Board Review Series

Surgical Specialties

Board Review Series

Surgical Specialties

Traves D. Crabtree, M.D.
Resident in General Surgery
Department of Surgery
University of Virginia
Charlottesville, Virginia

Associate Editors:

Eugene F. Foley, M.D.
Associate Professor of Surgery
Director of Colon & Rectal Surgery
Department of Surgery
University of Virginia
Charlottesville, Virginia

Robert G. Sawyer, M.D.
Assistant Professor of Surgery
Department of Surgery
University of Virginia
Charlottesville, Virginia

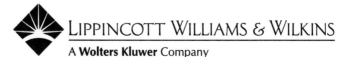

LIPPINCOTT WILLIAMS & WILKINS
A **Wolters Kluwer** Company
Philadelphia · Baltimore · New York · London
Buenos Aires · Hong Kong · Sydney · Tokyo

Editor: Elizabeth A. Nieginski
Editorial Director: Julie P. Martinez
Development Editors: Bridget Blatteau, Dvora Konstant
Marketing Manager: Aimee Sirmon
Managing Editor: Darrin Kiessling

351 West Camden Street
Baltimore, Maryland 21201-2436 USA

530 Walnut Street
Philadelphia, Pennsylvania 19106 USA

Printed in the United States of America

Library of Congress Cataloging-in-Publication Data

Surgical specialties / [edited by] Traves D. Crabtree ; associate editors, Eugene F. Foley, Robert G. Sawyer.
    p. ; cm. — (Board review series)
    Includes index.
    ISBN 0-7817-2771-5
    1. Surgery—Examinations, questions, etc. I. Crabtree, Traves D. II. Foley, Eugene F. III. Sawyer, Robert G. IV. Series.
    [DNLM: 1. Surgical Procedures, Operative—Examination Questions. WO 18.2 S9619 2000]
    RD37.2.S98 2000
    617'.0076—dc21

                                                                00-025010

To purchase additional copies of this book call our customer service department at **(800) 638-3030** or fax orders to **(301) 824-7390**. International customers should call **(301) 714-2324**.

                                            00 01 02
                                    1 2 3 4 5 6 7 8 9

Contents

Preface

BRS Surgical Specialties is designed as a companion text to *BRS General Surgery.* Like its counterpart, *BRS Surgical Specialties* reviews topics that allow for successful performance on the surgical section of the United States Medical Licensing Examination (USMLE) Step 2.

BRS Surgical Specialties provides a comprehensive review of the surgical specialties. Organized by body system, it covers the epidemiology, pathogenesis, diagnosis, and treatment of major disorders in each area. It is designed to provide an understanding of the details of each disease process, but intentionally focuses on the practical clinical approach to diagnosis and management of surgical problems.

Instead of relying solely on standard text, we have used the outline format, in addition to numerous figures and tables, to present the essential concepts. We have also incorporated a self-examination feature that consists of numerous questions and explanations at the end of each chapter, in addition to a comprehensive examination at the end of the book.

Recognizing that no one style of presentation is appropriate for all students or all topics, we have incorporated input from a diverse group of experts. By doing so, we are hopeful that this text will supplement *BRS General Surgery* and provide an interesting, effective, and enjoyable review of the surgical specialties.

Contributors

Tord D. Alden, M.D.
Chief Resident
Department of Neurosurgery
University of Virginia
Charlottesville, Virginia

Ken R. Barba, M.D.
Resident
Department of Ophthalmology
Loyola University Medical Center
Maywood, Illinois

Victor M. Brugh III, M.D.
Resident
Department of Urology
University of Virginia
Charlottesville, Virginia

R. Cartland Burns, M.D.
Assistant Professor of Surgery and Pediatrics
Division of Pediatric Surgery
University of Virginia
Charlottesville, Virginia

Terence N. Chapman, M.D.
Resident
Department of Urology
University of Virginia
Charlottesville, Virginia

Abhinav Chhabra, M.D.
Resident
Department of Orthopaedic Surgery
University of Virginia
Charlottesville, Virginia

David Dorofi, M.D.
Resident
Department of Otolaryngology
University of Virginia
Charlottesville, Virginia

Brant R. Fulmer, M.D.
Resident
Department of Urology
University of Virginia
Charlottesville, Virginia

John A. Jane Jr., M.D.
Resident
Department of Neurosurgery
University of Virginia
Charlottesville, Virginia

Jeffrey J. Laurent, M.D.
Resident
Department of Neurosurgery
University of Virginia
Charlottesville, Virginia

Todd A. Milbrandt, M.D.
Resident
Department of Orthopaedic Surgery
University of Virginia
Charlottesville, Virginia

Patrick E. Parrino, M.D.
Resident in General Surgery
University of Virginia
Charlottesville, Virginia

Scott D. Ross, M.D.
Resident in General Surgery
University of Virginia
Charlottesville, Virginia

Jonas M. Sheehan, M.D.
Resident
Department of Neurosurgery
University of Virginia
Charlottesville, Virginia

1
Vascular

Scott D. Ross

I. Atherosclerosis

A. Pathophysiology

1. **Atherosclerosis**

—is a disease of the **intima** of large arteries.

—causes luminal narrowing, thrombosis, and occlusion associated with **ischemia of the end organ.**

2. **Atherosclerotic lesions**

a. **Fatty streaks**

—are subintimal collections of foam cells (lipid-filled smooth muscle cells or macrophages).

b. **Fibrous plaques**

—are advanced lesions characterized by a thick fibrous luminal cap containing smooth muscle cells and leukocytes overlying a central core of necrotic debris and lipid (the atheroma).

c. **Complicated plaques**

—develop ulceration, luminal thrombosis, calcification, and wall hemorrhage.

B. Risk factors include

—cigarette smoking.

—hypertension.

—hypercholesterolemia.

—diabetes mellitus.

—hereditary factors.

C. Clinical sequelae of atherosclerosis

—depend on the location of the lesion (**Figure 1.1**).

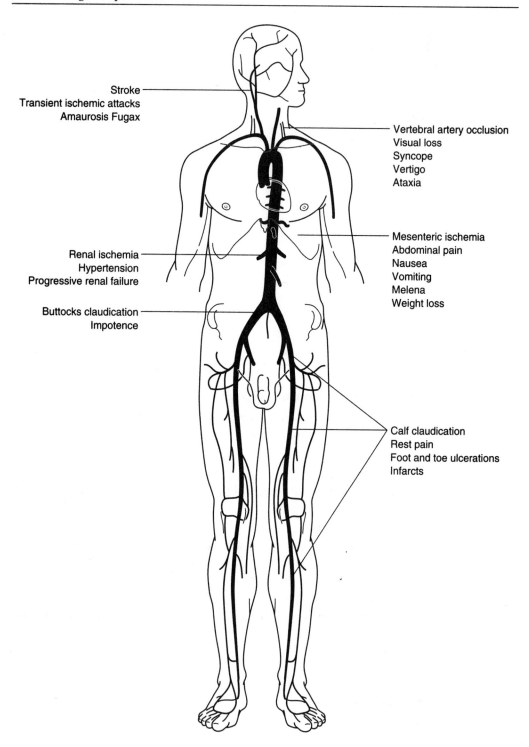

Stroke
Transient ischemic attacks
Amaurosis Fugax

Vertebral artery occlusion
Visual loss
Syncope
Vertigo
Ataxia

Mesenteric ischemia
Abdominal pain
Nausea
Vomiting
Melena
Weight loss

Renal ischemia
Hypertension
Progressive renal failure

Buttocks claudication
Impotence

Calf claudication
Rest pain
Foot and toe ulcerations
Infarcts

Figure 1.1. Clinical manifestations of arterial occlusive disease.

1. **Common types of arterial atherosclerosis** include

   —coronary.

   —carotid.

   —peripheral.

2. **Peripheral atherosclerosis may result in** different levels of symptoms ranging from intermittent claudication to foot pain to gangrene.

   —The level of symptomatology impacts treatment options in affected patients.

   a. **Claudication**

      —is profound fatigue, aching, or crampy pain in the extremity that is caused by exertion.

      —is **reproducible at a constant distance.**

      —is typically promptly **relieved by rest.**

   b. **Ischemic rest pain**

      —is intense pain, burning, or tingling **at rest,** usually across the distal foot and arch.

   c. **Gangrene** (tissue necrosis)

      —occurs when blood flow is inadequate to maintain tissue viability.

      —results in ischemic ulcers at distal tips or between the toes.

3. **Symptoms are caused by**

   —gradual progressive stenosis from an enlarging plaque.

   —sudden occlusion that is due to thrombosis of the vessel.

4. **Clinical sequelae**

   —are much more severe with sudden occlusion, which does not allow the development of collateral arterial channels.

II. Vascular Diagnostics

A. **Noninvasive studies**

1. **Ankle-brachial index (ABI)**

   —is the ankle systolic blood pressure divided by the brachial blood pressure with the patient in the **supine position.**

   a. **Normal average:** about 1.1.

   b. **Claudication:** average values of 0.6.

   c. **Rest pain:** mean ABI typically 0.25.

   d. **Impending gangrene:** ABIs seldom exceed 0.2 and average 0.05.

   e. **Incompressible arteries** from calcification (diabetes or renal failure) result in spuriously high values.

2. **Pulse volume recordings**

   —are performed by applying air-filled cuffs to the thigh, calf, and ankle.

   —Volume changes in soft tissue during pulsatile blood flow are recorded, thus providing information regarding the location of the disease.

3. **Duplex scanning**

—measures arterial obstruction by determining blood flow characteristics and velocity.

4. **Helical computed tomography (CT) and magnetic resonance (MR) angiography**

—provide multiple views of the vasculature.

B. **Diagnostic arterial angiography**

—remains the gold standard for vascular imaging.

1. The **overall rate of serious complications** is less than 2%.

2. **Complications** include

—hematoma.

—arterial dissection.

—pseudoaneurysm.

—arteriovenous fistula.

—thrombosis.

—embolism.

—renal failure.

—fluid overload.

—anaphylactoid reactions.

III. Acute Limb Ischemia

A. **Overview**

—Of acute arterial emboli, **80%–90% originate in the heart.**

1. **Other sites include**

—arterial aneurysms.

—peripheral arterial or aortic atherosclerotic plaques.

—sites of vascular trauma (including vascular catheterization).

2. **Two thirds of thrombi** of the heart arise secondary to **atrial fibrillation.** Other causes include

—acute myocardial infarction.

—left ventricular aneurysm with a mural thrombus.

—endocarditis.

—prosthetic heart valves (mitral valve most common).

—cardiac tumor (myxoma).

3. **Chronic atrial fibrillation**

—carries an annual risk of thromboembolic complications of 3%–6%.

4. **Paradoxical emboli,** which can cause stroke, are venous emboli that pass into the arterial system through defects connecting the right and left heart chambers (e.g., patent foramen ovale).

    5. Effective therapies

       —reduce thromboembolic complications.

       —include chronic warfarin therapy and possibly aspirin.

B. Clinical manifestations

    1. The **6 P's of peripheral ischemia** include

       —**pain** (severe, deep, well-localized, unremitting).

       —**pallor** (appears early).

       —**pulselessness.**

       —**paresthesia** (loss of light touch sensation in "stocking" or "glovelike" distribution).

       —**paralysis** (late feature).

       —**poikilothermia** (loss of temperature control–decreased temperature).

    2. Signs of impending irreversible limb ischemia include

       —complete loss of sensation.

       —diffuse mottling of the skin.

       —involuntary muscle contraction.

       —Loss of light touch sensation precedes loss of pain, pressure, and temperature sensation.

C. Differential diagnosis of acute limb ischemia includes

    —arterial embolism.

    —arterial thrombosis.

    —aortic wall dissection.

    —venous thrombosis.

    —arterial spasm.

    1. Characteristics differentiating arterial embolism from thrombosis are outlined in **Table 1-1.**

    2. With venous thrombosis

       —the onset of pain is more gradual.

Table 1-1. Distinctions Between Acute Arterial Embolism and Acute Arterial Thrombosis

Embolism	Thrombosis
Arrhythmia	No arrhythmia
Sudden onset	Sudden onset
No prior claudication or rest pain	History of claudication or rest pain
Normal contralateral pulses	Contralateral pulses absent
No physical findings of chronic limb ischemia	Physical findings of chronic limb ischemia

—the skin is somewhat darker, with prominent venous distension.

—swelling is common.

3. **If the diagnosis is in doubt,** duplex scanning or angiography should be performed.

D. Management of acute arterial insufficiency

—of the extremity must include rapid diagnosis and prompt correction of the occlusion.

1. Patients should be **immediately heparinized** when the clinical diagnosis is made.

2. **Contraindications to heparin** include

—a new neurologic deficit.

—gastrointestinal bleeding.

—other potential sites of bleeding.

3. **Early angiography**

—allows for anatomic localization of the occlusion.

—provides clues to the etiology (e.g., emboli versus thrombotic event).

—may occasionally play a role in treatment (e.g., tissue plasminogen activator).

4. If there is any question about the **viability of the limb,** surgical extraction of the thrombus (**thromboembolectomy**) should be considered for emboli disease.

—Bypass of the occluded segments may be necessary in some situations.

5. **Fasciotomy** to relieve compartmental pressure and avoid compression of arterial and venous vessels should be considered when ischemia lasts for more than 4 hours.

6. **Nonsurgical therapy** includes thrombolytic therapy through a catheter placed angiographically as close to the clot as possible.

7. **Complications of reperfusion of ischemic tissue** include

—lactic acidosis.

—hyperkalemia.

—myoglobinuria or acute tubular necrosis.

—muscle edema or compartment syndrome.

E. Atheroembolism

—is the sudden rupture of an atherosclerotic plaque, resulting in showers of atheromatous debris into the distal arterial circulation.

1. **Atheroembolism may occur**

—spontaneously.

—by surgical manipulation of the aorta or its major branches.

—by catheter manipulation during angiography.

2. **"Blue toe syndrome"**

—is lower extremity atheroembolism, manifested by sharply demarcated areas of focal ischemia of the lower leg or foot, typically in the toes.

a. **Symptoms** include

—**intense pain.**

—**purplish discoloration** of the skin and surrounding petechial hemorrhages.

—**thigh and calf myalgias.**

b. These **patients typically** have palpable distal pulses.

c. **Management**

(1) **Arteriography and echocardiography**

—delineate possible sources of emboli.

(2) **Surgical therapy**

—involves **endarterectomy,** excision, and bypass and exclusion of the diseased portion of the vessel.

(3) **Heparin**

—is also frequently used in the treatment of this disease.

3. **Lumbar sympathectomy**

—is rarely used but can be an adjunct to help increase cutaneous circulation in patients with severe refractory disease.

4. **Other clinical syndromes include**

—gastrointestinal microembolism.

—renal atheroembolism.

IV. Cerebrovascular Occlusive Disease

A. **Overview**

1. **Stroke** (cerebrovascular accident)

—remains the third most common cause of death in the United States.

2. **Carotid artery atherosclerosis**

—is the most common cause of stroke.

3. **Anatomy (Figure 1.2)**

a. **The paired internal carotid arteries**

—provide 80%–90% of total cerebral blood flow.

b. The **vertebral arteries**

—supply 10%–20% of cerebral flow.

c. The **circle of Willis**

—connects the anterior and posterior circulations.

B. **Pathophysiology**

1. The **carotid bifurcation**

—is the most common site of disease in the cerebral circulation.

2. **Ischemia**

—results from atheromatous emboli from a plaque.

—also occurs because of low flow distal to the stenosis, most commonly at a "watershed" area between the anterior and posterior circulation.

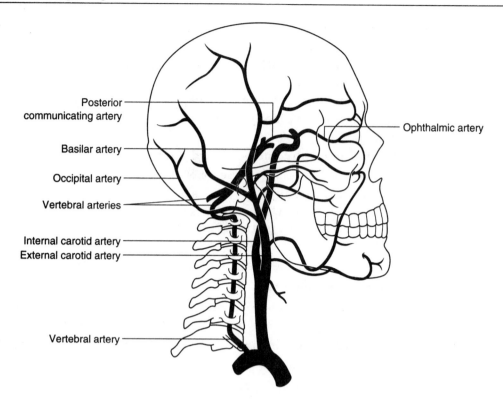

Figure 1.2. The arterial blood supply to the brain. (Adapted with permission from Greenfield L, Mulholland, Oldham, et al: *Surgery: Scientific Principles and Practice,* 2nd ed. Baltimore, Lippincott Williams & Wilkins, 1997, p 1748.)

C. Clinical presentation (Table 1-2)

    1. Transient ischemic attack (TIA)

        —is the sudden onset of a focal neurologic deficit that resolves completely **within 24 hours** of its onset.

        a. Transient hemispheric ischemic attacks

            —involve sudden onset of contralateral motor and/or sensory deficits.

        b. Amaurosis fugax

            —is transient loss of vision in the ipsilateral eye, secondary to obstruction of branch of ophthalmic artery.

    2. Vertebrobasilar insufficiency results in

        —binocular visual loss.

        —drop attacks.

        —dysarthria.

        —vertigo.

        —dysphasia.

        —incoordination.

    3. Stroke

        —is an acute onset of neurologic symptoms that continues for more than

Table 1-2. Symptoms of Cerebrovascular Occlusive Disease

Syndrome	Clinical Presentation	Duration of Symptoms
Transient ischemic attack	Sudden onset of contralateral motor and/or sensory deficits	< 24 hours
Amaurosis fugax	Transient loss of vision in ipsilateral eye	< 24 hours
Vertebrobasilar insufficiency	Dizziness, vertigo, dysphagia, drop attacks	May be < or > 24 hours
Stroke	Permanent neurologic deficit and nonviable brain tissue	> 24 hours

24 hours. The symptoms are caused by ischemia (i.e., emboli or thrombi) or hemorrhage within or around the brain.

    a. Middle cerebral artery territory occlusion results in
        —contralateral hemiparesis or hemiplegia.
        —paralysis of contralateral lower part of the face.
        —contralateral homonymous hemianopsia (visual field deficit).
        —aphasia.

    b. Anterior cerebral artery territory blockage causes
        —contralateral monoplegia.
        —sparing of face.
        —abnormalities of higher cerebral function.

D. Diagnosis

    1. Physical examination
        —distinguishes between a focal and a nonfocal neurologic deficit.

    2. Noninvasive color-flow duplex scanning
        —is characteristically used to identify the degree of carotid stenosis.

    3. Angiography
        —Carotid angiography is associated with a 1%–2% risk of stroke.

    4. CT scan
        —distinguishes between cerebral **hemorrhage and infarction.**
        —within the first 24 hours will identify hemorrhage but may not demonstrate an area of infarction.

    5. MR imaging
        —can detect a stroke immediately after the infarction occurs.
        —is rapidly becoming the test of choice for evaluation of acute onset of cerebrovascular occlusive events.

E. Management

1. **Medical therapy**

—is for prevention and treatment of sequelae of cerebrovascular disease.

a. **Modification of risk factors**

—particularly **hypertension,** is important to prevent progression of disease. Cessation of smoking, lowering cholesterol, and controlling diabetes are also important.

b. **Aspirin**

—has been shown to reduce the risk of stroke and death in patients with documented cerebrovascular disease.

(1) Systemic anticoagulation with warfarin may be beneficial.

(2) **Ticlopidine** may also be used when aspirin is contraindicated.

c. **Systemic anticoagulation and thrombolytic therapy**

—may be beneficial in certain patients with ischemic stroke.

—should not be administered to patients with a hemorrhagic stroke.

2. **Indications for surgical therapy**

a. **Symptomatic patients**

—with recent TIAs or nondisabling strokes and an ipsilateral high-grade carotid stenosis of **60%–99%** are indicated for surgical therapy.

—The 2-year risk of ipsilateral stroke in surgical patients is 9%, but it is 26% in patients receiving medical therapy alone.

b. **Asymptomatic patients**

—with internal carotid artery stenosis of **60%–99%** benefit from surgery.

—Overall, the 2-year risk of ipsilateral stroke in surgically treated, asymptomatic patients is 5%, versus 10% in patients receiving medical therapy only.

—The decrease in the incidence of stroke with surgery may be more pronounced in men when compared to the decrease seen in women.

3. **Carotid endarterectomy (CEA)**

—removes the atherosclerotic plaques that occupy the media and intima of the diseased vessel.

a. **Structures encountered during a carotid endarterectomy** are outlined in **Figure 1.3.**

b. **Complications of carotid endarterectomy**

(1) **Stroke** or transient cerebral ischemia (1%–2%)

(2) **Cranial nerve injury** (e.g., recurrent laryngeal, hypoglossal, and superior laryngeal)

(3) **Bleeding**

(4) **Myocardial infarction,** which is the most common source of non-stroke-related morbidity and mortality

(5) **Postoperative hypertension,** resulting from degeneration of the carotid body

V. Mesenteric Vascular Disease

A. **Vascular anatomy of the abdominal viscera**

1. The **celiac artery** gives rise to the splenic artery, the **proper hepatic** artery, and the left gastric artery.

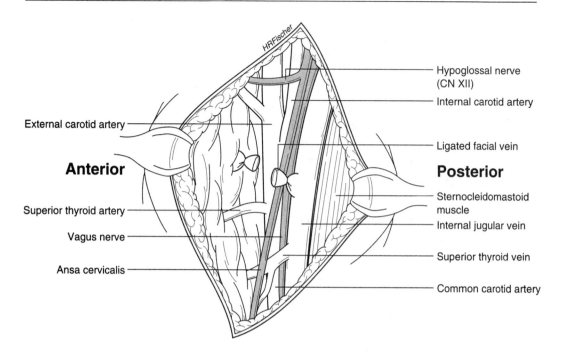

External carotid artery

Anterior

Superior thyroid artery

Vagus nerve

Ansa cervicalis

HRFischer

Hypoglossal nerve
(CN XII)

Internal carotid artery

Ligated facial vein

Posterior

Sternocleidomastoid
muscle

Internal jugular vein

Superior thyroid vein

Common carotid artery

Figure 1.3. Anatomic structures encountered during a left carotid endarterectomy (CEA). The recurrent laryngeal nerve runs deep to the vagus nerve between the carotid artery and the internal jugular vein. (Adapted from Blackbourne L, Fleischer KJ: *Advanced Surgical Recall.* Baltimore, Lippincott Williams & Wilkins, 1997, p 787.)

2. The **superior mesenteric artery (SMA) provides arterial blood supply to the**

—pancreas.

—small intestine.

—ascending and right half of the transverse colon.

3. The **inferior mesenteric artery (IMA) provides arterial blood supply to**

—the left half of the transverse colon.

—all of the descending colon.

4. The **marginal artery of Drummond and arc of Riolan**

—are important sources of collateral blood supply between the SMA and IMA.

B. Acute mesenteric ischemia

1. Mesenteric embolism and mesenteric thrombosis

—account for the majority of cases of acute mesenteric ischemia.

a. Nonocclusive mesenteric ischemia that results from a low-flow state, such as cardiogenic shock, is another etiology.

b. Mesenteric venous thrombosis may also cause acute mesenteric ischemia.

2. Clinical presentation

a. Sudden onset of pain, severe epigastric or mid-abdominal, is followed promptly by evacuation of the gut, either through emesis or explosive diarrhea.

b. Abdominal examination may reveal signs of peritonitis or may be normal.

c. Severe abdominal complaints out of proportion to the physical findings is a well-recognized early presentation.

d. Peritoneal signs or blood in the stool are late, ominous signs, implying severe ischemia with infarction.

—Associated mortality is 70%.

3. Diagnosis

—The diagnosis is frequently based on clinical suspicion followed by emergent **angiography.**

—Late findings may include hemoconcentration, acidosis, and leukocytosis.

4. Treatment

a. Initial measures include

—heparin, volume resuscitation, and antibiotics.

b. Emergent surgical intervention

—may involve embolectomy or bypass of the diseased vessel and bowel resection if necrosis has occurred.

c. Assessment of intestinal viability

(1) Clinical parameters of color, spontaneous peristalsis, and the presence or absence of **palpable pulses** are often used to assess bowel viability.

(2) Intraoperative Doppler ultrasound of the vessels or administration of fluorescein dye, which localizes in viable tissue, may also be used.

(3) A second-look procedure in 24–48 hours is frequently performed to reassess for potentially nonviable intestine that requires resection.

d. Overall **mortality** is 70% or higher.

C. Chronic mesenteric ischemia

1. Visceral angina

—is secondary to arteriosclerotic disease that is typically widespread throughout the mesenteric arcades.

a. Symptoms include

—midepigastric pain 30–45 minutes after eating.

—weight loss from avoidance of food secondary to pain.

b. Diagnosis

—is made with **arteriography.**

c. Treatment

—involves removal of the plaque (endarterectomy) or arterial bypass of the diseased segments.

2. Mesenteric venous thrombosis may be secondary to

—intra-abdominal inflammatory processes.

—portal hypertension.

—hypercoagulable states.

—the use of oral contraceptives.

  a. **Symptoms**

  —include a vague prodrome of crampy abdominal pain, abdominal distension, nausea and malaise.

  b. **Diagnosis**

  —**CT scan may demonstrate thrombus within the portal vein** or superior mesenteric vein.

  —The diagnosis, however, is usually made intraoperatively.

  c. **Treatment** consists of

  —resection of nonviable intestine.

  —thrombolytic therapy.

  —occasional large vessel venous thrombectomy.

  —the use of anticoagulants.

  —correction of any predisposing cause or hypercoagulable state.

VI. Renal Artery Occlusive Disease

A. Pathophysiology of renovascular hypertension

  1. Renal artery stenosis

  —reduces renal perfusion.

  —**increases renin release** from the juxtaglomerular apparatus.

  2. Renin

  —stimulates conversion of angiotensinogen to angiotensin, which leads to increased aldosterone release accounting for the **elevated blood pressure** (see *BRS General Surgery,* Chapter 20 II B 2)

  3. The most common causes are

  —**atherosclerosis,** which is typically bilateral.

  —**arterial fibrodysplasia (medial fibroplasia fibromuscular dysplasia** is seen most frequently in **young women).**

B. Clinical features of renovascular hypertension

  1. Systolic and diastolic **upper abdominal bruits**

  2. Diastolic blood pressures over 115 mm Hg

  3. Sudden worsening of mild to moderate essential hypertension

  4. Development of hypertension during childhood

  5. Rapid onset of high blood pressure after the age of 50 years

  6. Hypertension resistant to drug therapy

C. Diagnosis

  —can occasionally be made by renal artery ultrasound, but arteriography or MR angiography are used most frequently.

D. Treatment

  1. Drug therapy to control hypertension is often successful in the initial management.

    a. **Angiotensin-converting enzyme (ACE) inhibitors** (e.g., lisinopril, captopril)

      —are frequently effective.

      —may, however, cause a critical decrease in intrarenal blood pressure with renal ischemia.

    b. **Angiotensin II receptor antagonists** (e.g., losartan)

      —may also be used to control hypertension in this setting.

2. **Percutaneous transluminal renal angioplasty and possible stent placement** are most effective in the treatment of lesions in the mid-portion of the renal artery.

   —Angioplasty of **atherosclerotic stenoses** may be limited by an inability to dilate the spillover plaque (ostial lesions) from extensive aortic disease.

3. **Renal revascularization and endarterectomy** are options for surgical therapy.

   —**Endarterectomy** is often the preferred means of treating proximal renal artery atherosclerotic disease.

   —The **poorest response** to surgery is noted in those patients with generalized atherosclerosis.

4. **Nephrectomy** is an alternative in patients with a unilateral vascular lesion and a normal contralateral kidney.

VII. Aortoiliac Occlusive Disease

A. Pathophysiology

1. **Arteriosclerosis**

   —can produce partial or complete occlusion of the aorta and iliac arteries (the inflow vessels) (**Figure 1.4**).

2. The **disease process** is commonly centered around the aortic bifurcation.

B. Clinical symptoms

1. **Claudication**

   —may involve the proximal musculature of the thigh, hip, or buttock area.

2. **Complete occlusion of the distal aorta (i.e., Leriche syndrome)** may be associated with

   —diminished femoral pulses.

   —buttock and thigh claudication.

   —impotence secondary to hypogastric arterial obstruction and reduction of blood flow through the internal pudendal artery.

C. Indications for operation

1. **Ischemic pain** at rest

2. **Tissue necrosis**

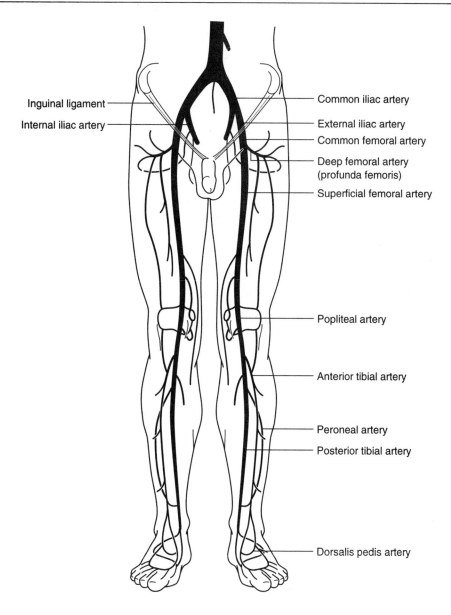

Inguinal ligament

Internal iliac artery

Common iliac artery

External iliac artery

Common femoral artery

Deep femoral artery
(profunda femoris)

Superficial femoral artery

Popliteal artery

Anterior tibial artery

Peroneal artery

Posterior tibial artery

Dorsalis pedis artery

Figure 1.4. The lower extremity arterial circulation.

3. Claudication, which jeopardizes the livelihood of a patient or significantly impairs the lifestyle of an otherwise low-risk patient

4. Distal **atheromatous embolization** from proximal aortoiliac disease

D. Operative procedures (Figure 1.5)

1. Aortobifemoral bypass grafting

—from the infrarenal aorta to femoral arteries is an effective method of revascularization.

a. The proximal anastomosis

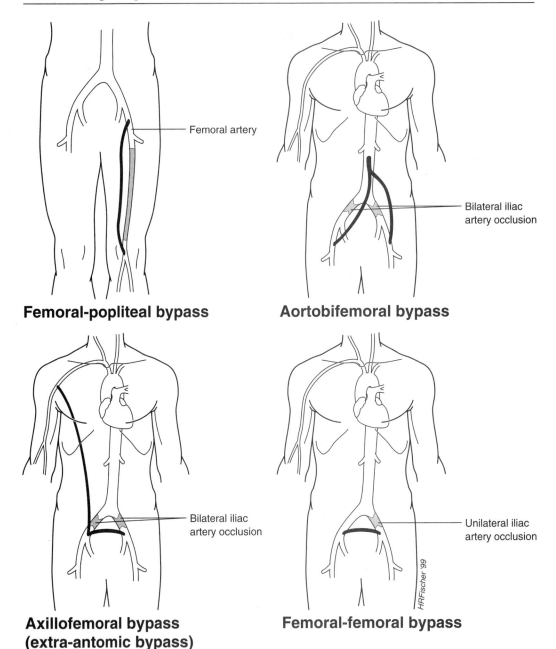

Femoral-popliteal bypass — Femoral artery

Aortobifemoral bypass — Bilateral iliac artery occlusion

Axillofemoral bypass (extra-antomic bypass) — Bilateral iliac artery occlusion

Femoral-femoral bypass — Unilateral iliac artery occlusion

HRFischer '99

Figure 1.5. Arterial bypass procedures used in patients with arterial occlusive disease. (Adapted with permission from Lawrence P: *Essentials of General Surgery,* 2nd ed. Baltimore, Williams & Wilkins, 1992, p 335.)

—is placed as high as possible on the infrarenal aorta where there is a lesser amount of disease.

b. **The distal anastomosis**

—is constructed at the femoral level, often establishing adequate graft outflow through the profunda femoris artery.

c. **Perioperative mortality** is less than 5%.

—Five-year graft patency rates approach 85%–90%.

   d. Femofemoral and Iliofemoral bypass grafts

   —may be useful for patients with disease confined to the external iliac artery of one extremity.

2. Axillofemoral and femorofemoral bypass grafts

   a. These **extra-anatomic grafts** are routed in subcutaneous tissue planes to

   —avoid hostile pathologic conditions around the aorta (e.g., **bacterial infection,** multiple previous operations).

   —decrease the risk of operation associated with laparotomy in high-risk patients.

   b. These grafts, however, have lower patency rates when compared with aortic grafts.

3. Aortoiliac endarterectomy

   —may be used for localized atherosclerotic disease confined to the distal aorta, aortic bifurcation, and common iliac arteries.

VIII. Femoropopliteal and Infrapopliteal Occlusive Disease

A. Anatomy (see **Figure 1.4**)

1. The common femoral artery begins at the inguinal ligament as the direct extension of the external iliac artery.

   a. The **common femoral artery divides into**

   —the more lateral and posterior **deep femoral artery (i.e., the profunda femoris).**

   —the more medial **superficial femoral artery.**

   b. The superficial femoral artery

   —is the artery in the leg most likely to be obstructed by atherosclerosis.

2. The popliteal artery

   a. This artery is a continuation of the superficial femoral artery, which emerges from the adductor (Hunter) canal and proceeds posteriorly behind the knee.

   b. Its branches include

   —the **anterior tibial artery,** which terminates in the foot as the dorsalis pedis artery.

   —the **posterior tibial** and **peroneal** arteries.

B. Clinical presentation

1. Intermittent claudication, typically affecting the calf

2. Ischemic rest pain of the forefoot and toes

3. Ischemic ulcers and **gangrene** of the distal toes and forefoot

   —In contrast, **ulcers** secondary to venous insufficiency often occur over the medial malleolus.

   a. Wet gangrene represents necrosis with infection and purulence.

      b. Dry gangrene generally represents aseptic necrosis.

   4. Classic signs of lower extremity ischemia include

—pallor.

—hair loss.

—dependent rubor.

—abnormal nail growth.

—slow capillary filling.

C. Nonoperative treatment of lower extremity ischemia

   1. An exercise program

—of walking produces a predictable and significant improvement in symptoms of claudication.

   2. Risk factor modification

—particularly **cessation of smoking,** is essential.

   3. Cilostazol

—inhibits platelet aggregation and causes vasodilation to improve symptoms of claudication.

   4. Aspirin

—reduces the overall vascular mortality rate by 15%.

   5. Directed angiographic thrombolysis

—involves infusion of thrombolytic agents (**urokinase, tissue plasminogen activator**) near a thrombus.

—may be used for treatment of acute ischemia.

   6. Percutaneous transluminal angioplasty (PTA)

—is effective for localized, short stenoses in the iliac vessels but is inferior to surgical bypass in femoral popliteal disease.

—A balloon attached to an angiographic catheter is fluoroscopically guided to the occlusion and inflated to fracture the plaque and enlarge the arterial lumen.

D. Operative treatment of infrainguinal occlusive disease

   1. Indications for surgery include

—ischemic rest pain.

—tissue necrosis of leg or foot.

—claudication, which interferes significantly with employment or performance of daily tasks.

   2. Femoropopliteal bypass

—is performed for superficial femoral artery occlusion, using prosthetic grafts for anastomoses above the knee and autogenous saphenous vein for popliteal anastomoses below the knee.

—**Femorotibial artery bypass** is required for occlusive disease in the popliteal and tibial vessels.

a. **Complications** include

—myocardial infarction.

—wound complications.

b. **If a vein is not available,** or is not suitable for bypass, a prosthetic graft may be used.

—But patency rates are lower than those achieved with autogenous veins, especially in bypasses below the knee.

3. **Amputation should be considered**

—in patients who have limb ischemia from arterial obstructive disease that is so advanced that revascularization is not possible.

—in patients who have no potential for ambulation even after successful revascularization.

—in cases of systemic sepsis.

a. **The level of amputation**

—should be below the knee if possible to allow for the greatest chance of rehabilitation.

b. **The long-term mortality** after amputation

—for vascular disease is 50% at 3 years and 70% at 5 years, frequently because of comorbid conditions.

IX. Nonatherosclerotic Vascular Disease

A. **Thromboangiitis obliterans (Buerger disease)**

1. **Overview**

—This typically affects **young male smokers** (20–35 years old).

—This disease is **characterized by** transmural inflammation of small and medium-sized arteries.

2. **Signs and symptoms** include

—**severe rest pain with bilateral ulceration.**

—gangrene of the digits, particularly the fingers.

3. **Treatment**

—**Primary treatment** involves cessation of **tobacco use.**

—**Sympathectomy** may provide some benefit in patients with refractory disease, although amputation is frequently required with progression of disease.

B. **Takayasu's arteritis** (rare)

1. **Overview**

—This usually affects **young Asian women** (younger than 30 years old).

—This type of arteritis is **characterized by inflammation of large vessels** (aorta, aortic arch vessels, pulmonary arteries).

2. **Symptoms**

—include fever, arthralgia, myalgia, and anorexia.

3. Primary treatment

—is with **high-dose steroids.**

4. Complications

—include stroke, hypertension, and congestive heart failure.

X. Aneurysmal Disease

A. Thoracic aortic aneurysms

1. Etiologies

—include **cystic medial necrosis** associated with Marfan's syndrome, **atherosclerosis,** and **trauma.**

2. Symptoms

—**are secondary** to compression or obstruction of adjacent structures, dissection, or rupture.

a. **Classic symptoms** are chest and **back pain.**

b. **Voice change** occurs because of left recurrent laryngeal nerve compression.

c. **Tracheobronchial obstruction** causes cough or dyspnea.

d. **Esophageal obstruction** causes dysphagia.

e. **Dilation of the aortic root** may result in **aortic regurgitation** and heart failure.

3. Diagnosis

a. **Chest radiograph**

—may show a mediastinal mass continuous with the aortic shadow.

b. **CT scan**

c. **Aortography** of the arch and descending thoracic aorta

4. Management

a. **Surgical graft replacement**

—is the treatment of choice.

(1) **Emergent surgical repair** is indicated for patients with **symptomatic aneurysms or rupture,** regardless of size.

(2) **Elective repair** is indicated for good-risk asymptomatic patients with aneurysms larger than 5.5–6.0 cm in diameter.

(3) **Patients with Marfan's syndrome** or aortic dissection are generally treated more aggressively.

b. **Complications**

(1) **Operative mortality** (5%–10%)

(2) **Myocardial dysfunction**

(3) **Hemorrhage**

(4) **Paraplegia,** which may develop from spinal cord ischemia caused by occlusion of critical intercostal arteries and the **artery of Adamkiewicz** during the repair

(5) **Renal ischemia** and **renal failure**

B. Abdominal aortic aneurysms (AAAs)

1. An aneurysm

—is a permanent localized dilation of an artery to 1.5 times or more its normal diameter (normal infrarenal aorta = 2.0 cm).

2. **Classification**

   —is described in **Figure 1.6.**

3. **Clinical manifestations**

   a. **Infrarenal AAAs**

   —Seventy to seventy five percent are **asymptomatic** when diagnosed.

   (1) **Symptoms** may be **caused by**

   —rupture or expansion.

   —pressure on adjacent structures.

   —distal embolism.

   —dissection.

   (2) **Abdominal or back pain** is the most common symptom.

   b. **Ruptured AAA**

   (1) **Wall tension**

   —is directly related to intraluminal pressure and radius (law of Laplace).

   (2) **Rupture of an AAA classically presents with**

   —**abdominal or back pain.**

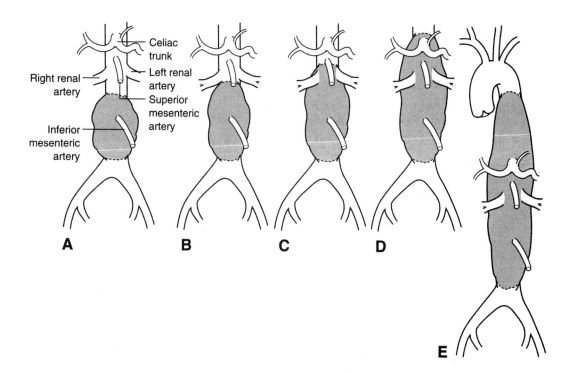

Figure 1.6. Classification of abdominal aortic aneurysms. (*A*) Infrarenal (*B*) Juxtarenal (*C*) Pararenal (*D*) Suprarenal (*E*) Thoracoabdominal. (Adapted from Greenfield L, Mulholland, Oldham, et al: *Surgery: Scientific Principles and Practice,* 2nd ed. Baltimore, Lippincott, Williams & Wilkins, 1997, p 1882.)

—syncopal or near-syncopal episodes.

—**shock.**

—a **pulsatile abdominal mass.**

(3) **Risk of aneurysm rupture** (5-year rupture rates)

(a) Aneurysm smaller than 4 cm are unlikely to rupture

(b) Aneurysm 5–7 cm ≈ 33%

(c) Aneurysm larger than 7 cm > 80%

4. **Diagnostic methods**

a. **Physical examination**

—The **expansile** nature of a **pulsatile mass** is the key element in deciding whether a palpable abdominal mass is an aneurysm.

b. **Ultrasound**

—is the modality of choice for initial evaluation and follow-up to determine increase in size.

c. **CT scan**

—accurately measures the size and extent of the aneurysm.

d. **Aortography**

—is used to define the extent of aneurysm formation, especially suprarenal and iliac involvement, and to determine run-off in the legs in patients with claudication or poor distal pulses.

—cannot be relied on to determine the diameter of an aneurysm or even to establish its presence because of the mural thrombus.

5. **Indications for emergent surgical intervention**

a. **Known or suspected rupture,** regardless of the size of the aneurysm or the patient's age

b. **Symptomatic aneurysms** without signs of rupture

6. **Indications for elective operation**

a. **Aneurysms larger than 5 cm in diameter** in **asymptomatic** patients who are acceptable operative risks

b. **Aneurysms 4–5 cm in diameter** in good-risk patients

c. **Rapid expansion of the aneurysm by more than 0.4 cm in diameter per year**

7. **Aneurysms are usually repaired surgically** by **replacing the diseased segment** of aorta with a prosthetic graft.

a. **IMA reimplantation**

—may be required to avoid infarction of the left colon if collateral blood flow to the bowel is inadequate.

b. **When an AAA is ruptured**

—the first priority is to **clamp the aorta above the site of rupture** (gain proximal control) to control hemorrhage.

8. **Complications**

a. Emergent surgery for a rupture, which is associated with a 50% perioperative mortality

b. Myocardial dysfunction

c. Hemorrhage

    d. Renal failure

    e. Ischemia of the left colon and rectum (about 2% of repairs), which typically presents with bloody diarrhea within 48 hours

    f. Lower extremity ischemia, which can be caused by embolism of dislodged mural thrombus, thrombosis of a vessel, or creation of an intimal flap

    g. Paraplegia from spinal cord ischemia, although this is a rare event after operations confined to the infrarenal aorta

    h. Infection of the prosthetic graft

        —A late complication associated with infection of prosthetic grafts is development of an **aortoenteric fistula** (gastrointestinal bleeding in a patient with a prosthetic graft in the abdomen).

    i. Disturbance of pelvic blood flow during repair, which may result in **impotence** and **disturbance of pelvic sympathetic nerves,** which may result in **retrograde ejaculation**

  9. New developments for treatment

    —include **endoluminal grafts,** vascular prostheses that are placed intraluminally using catheter-based deployment systems.

C. Other arterial aneurysms

  1. Iliac artery aneurysms often appear in continuity with AAAs.

    —Isolated iliac aneurysms are rare but should be treated surgically or with endovascular stents when they are discovered, to avoid the high mortality associated with rupture.

  2. Splenic artery aneurysms are the most common splanchnic artery aneurysms.

    a. They occur because of

      —medial fibrodysplasia.

      —**pregnancy.**

      —portal hypertension.

      —arterial disruptions due to adjacent inflammatory disease (e.g., **pancreatitis**).

    b. Signet-ring calcifications

      —are characteristic vascular calcifications seen on plain abdominal radiographs.

    c. Risk of rupture

      —is less than 2% in asymptomatic aneurysms.

      —is nearly 95% in aneurysms recognized during pregnancy.

      —also depends on the size of the aneurysm, with larger lesions (larger than 3 cm) at greater risk for rupture.

    d. Bleeding

      —may initially be contained within the lesser sac.

      —Free peritoneal hemorrhage eventually occurs causing shock (double-rupture phenomenon).

    e. Indications for repair include

      —**rupture.**

—**symptoms** (e.g., pain).

—the presence of an aneurysm in a **woman of childbearing age.**

3. **Femoral artery aneurysms** are commonly bilateral.

a. **Clinical manifestations** include

—local pain or the presence of a groin mass.

—lower extremity ischemia caused by thrombosis or distal embolization.

—compression of vein or nerve.

—rupture.

b. **Indications for operation** include

—**all symptomatic femoral aneurysms.**

—**asymptomatic aneurysms larger than 2.5 cm in diameter.**

c. The **femoral artery**

—is a common location of **pseudoaneurysms.**

(1) These are collections of blood in continuity with the arterial system but unenclosed by all three layers of the arterial wall.

(2) They may result from a disrupted suture line between a graft and the host artery, or from arterial wall defect created by **catheter insertion.**

(3) **Treatment** is with sonographic compression, with surgical repair required for lesions that are not adequately treated using this technique.

4. **Popliteal artery aneurysms** are the most common peripheral aneurysm.

a. **Bilateral aneurysms**

—are found in 50%–70% of patients.

—**AAAs are found in 70%** of these patients.

b. **Clinical manifestations** include

—limb ischemia usually from thrombosis.

—a **popliteal mass** and local pain or leg swelling from compression of adjacent neural or venous structures.

c. **Diagnosis**

—**Physical examination** detects prominent popliteal pulses.

—**Ultrasound** can visualize the aneurysm.

d. **Early surgical treatment**

—is recommended when popliteal aneurysm is diagnosed because of high incidence of complications.

—generally involves **ligation and bypass of the aneurysm.**

Review Test

Directions: Each of the numbered items or incomplete statements in this section is followed by answers or by completions of the statement. Select the ONE lettered answer or completion that is BEST in each case.

1. A 50-year-old man with a long history of buttock and thigh claudication presents with a 2-week history of pain in his left foot at rest. He underwent aortobifemoral bypass grafting 1 month ago and now presents with abdominal pain and fever. Computed tomography scan reveals a complex fluid collection near the bifurcation of the graft extending to the left groin. Which of the following is considered appropriate treatment for this patient?

(A) Oral antibiotics alone for 6 weeks and repeat angiography
(B) Intravenous antibiotics, removal of the entire prosthesis, and axillobifemoral bypass
(C) Surgical drainage of the left groin and oral antibiotics for 6 weeks
(D) Ligation of the left femoral artery and amputation if necessary
(E) Intravenous antibiotics and hospital observation

2. A 65-year-old man with a 50 pack-year smoking history (2 packs/day × 25 years) complains of recurring right calf pain after walking approximately 50 yards. This discomfort occurs only with activity, and resolves rapidly with rest. He has palpable femoral and pedal pulses. Which of the following is the next step in his diagnostic evaluation?

(A) Venous Doppler ultrasound
(B) Venogram
(C) Arteriography
(D) Duplex scanning
(E) Ankle-brachial indices

3. A 76-year-old woman presents with a 6-cm abdominal aortic aneurysm. She subsequently undergoes elective surgical repair of the aneurysm. Two days postoperatively, she has bloody diarrhea. Which of the following should be considered the most likely cause of this patient's symptoms?

(A) Aortoenteric fistula
(B) Ischemic colitis
(C) Pseudomembranous colitis
(D) Duodenal ischemia
(E) Stress gastritis

4. After aortic reconstruction for an abdominal aortic aneurysm, the surgeon is concerned about the development of ischemic colitis. Ischemic colitis can be diagnosed most reliably by

(A) Postoperative barium enema
(B) Intraoperative Doppler arterial signal in the sigmoid mesentery
(C) Intraoperative observation of bowel peristalsis
(D) Postoperative sigmoidoscopy
(E) Intraoperative measurement of inferior mesenteric artery stump pressure

5. A 70-year-old man presents to his family physician with complaints of pain behind his right knee. On physical examination, prominent popliteal pulses are noted and sharply demarcated areas of purplish discoloration of the skin are identified on the patient's foot. Ultrasound confirms the presence of a popliteal artery aneurysm. Which of the following is the next step in the management of this patient?

(A) Follow-up appointment in 1 year
(B) Anticoagulation therapy
(C) Ultrasound evaluation for abdominal aortic aneurysm
(D) Emergent surgical repair
(E) Angiography

6. A 55-year-old man is scheduled to undergo elective coronary artery bypass, and an asymptomatic right carotid bruit is discovered during evaluation. Which of the following statements is true regarding asymptomatic carotid bruits?

(A) Their detection mandates surgical intervention
(B) Their presence is a predictor of symptomatic coronary artery disease
(C) Their presence predicts the occurrence of stroke
(D) Their presence highly correlates with significant carotid stenosis
(E) Their presence has no clinical significance

7. A 60-year-old woman develops weakness in her right arm and she has some difficulty speaking. This condition resolves after 5 minutes, and she has no residual symptoms. No carotid bruit is heard on physical examination, and her electrocardiogram is normal. Which of the following is the next step in her evaluation?

(A) Performance of a stress thallium test
(B) Performance of a transesophageal echocardiogram
(C) Observation and initiation of aspirin therapy
(D) Observation and initiation of warfarin therapy
(E) Performance of a carotid duplex scan

8. A patient presents to his family physician with intermittent episodes of blindness in his right eye. He is found to have 80% carotid artery stenosis on the right and 85% stenosis of the contralateral carotid artery, which is asymptomatic. Which of the following is the appropriate initial treatment?

(A) Simultaneous bilateral carotid endarterectomy
(B) Carotid endarterectomy on the side with the greatest stenosis
(C) Carotid endarterectomy on the symptomatic side
(D) Staged bilateral endarterectomy with a 1-week interval between stages
(E) Percutaneous transluminal angioplasty of both carotids

9. A 65-year-old woman with a long history of atrial fibrillation presents to the emergency room with a history of sudden onset of severe abdominal pain that was followed by one episode of emesis. The physical examination is remarkable for the absence of peritoneal signs despite the patient's complaint of severe pain. Her past surgical history is significant for a vaginal hysterectomy. Which of the following is the most appropriate initial diagnostic procedure?

(A) Computed tomography (CT) scan to rule out complicated diverticulitis
(B) Nasogastric decompression, bowel rest, and observation
(C) Upper endoscopy to rule out duodenal ulcer
(D) Angiographic evaluation of mesenteric vessels
(E) Right upper quadrant ultrasound to rule out a biliary source

10. An otherwise healthy man presents for elective surgical repair of a 5.6-cm abdominal aortic aneurysm. During preoperative evaluation, the patient is found to have significant bilateral stenosis of the iliac arteries. He subsequently undergoes aortobifemoral bypass of the aneurysm and the stenotic areas. Which of the following complications occurs most commonly after such a repair in a 58-year-old man?

(A) Renal failure
(B) Impotence
(C) Ischemic colitis
(D) Leg paralysis
(E) Peripheral embolization

11. A 55-year-old man with a history of intermittent calf claudication develops a nonhealing ulcer of his lower extremity. Arteriography reveals occlusion of the superficial femoral artery with a reconstitution at the level of the popliteal artery. With regard to femoropopliteal bypass, which of the following statements is true?

(A) The patency of autologous vein grafts is better than with prosthetic grafts
(B) Continued cigarette smoking has no effect on graft patency
(C) Patency rates of femoropopliteal grafts are unaffected by vein size
(D) In situ vein bypass has better patency rates than reversed vein bypass
(E) Patency rates are unaffected by the indication for operation

12. A 45-year-old man, who suffered an acute myocardial infarction 5 months ago, presents to the emergency department with a painful, cool, and pulseless left lower extremity. He demonstrates loss of light touch sensation in his left foot. After undergoing femoral embolectomy and fasciotomy, he becomes oliguric, and his urine turns red. Immediate treatment includes

(A) Administration of intravenous (IV) fluids and reversal of heparin effects
(B) Administration of IV fluids and a 20 mEq potassium chloride bolus
(C) Administration of IV fluids, sodium bicarbonate, and mannitol
(D) Administration of IV fluids and immediate renal arteriography
(E) Immediate blood transfusion with cross-matched donor blood

13. A patient with a history of claudication continues to develop painful areas of purplish discoloration on the toes of both feet. Arteriography reveals diffuse atherosclerosis of the aortoiliac bifurcation, and he undergoes aortobifemoral bypass. Which of the following is the most common late graft-related complication of aortic bypass grafts?

(A) Graft occlusion from progressive atherosclerosis
(B) Pseudoaneurysm formation at the suture line
(C) Formation of an aortoenteric fistula
(D) Distal embolization from graft thrombus
(E) Graft infection caused by transient bacteremia

14. A patient with significant occlusive disease of the aortoiliac bifurcation developed ischemic pain in his lower extremities at rest. He underwent revascularization with aortobifemoral bypass graft and is recovering in the intensive care unit. Which of the following is the most common cause of death after recovery from successful aortic bypass graft?

(A) Rupture of pseudoaneurysm
(B) Acute graft thrombosis
(C) Coronary artery disease
(D) Cerebrovascular accident
(E) Renal failure

15. A 65-year-old man presents to his family physician and describes a brief loss of vision in one eye approximately 2 weeks ago. He denies any current visual changes. On physical examination, he does not have a carotid bruit but he does have an abnormal funduscopic examination. Occlusion of which of the following vessels is most likely associated with this patient's findings?

(A) Facial artery
(B) Occipital artery
(C) Vertebral artery
(D) Retinal artery
(E) Posterior auricular artery

16. A 55-year-old woman with a history of insulin-dependent diabetes mellitus, hypertension, and 3 days of fever and chills presents to the emergency room with a fever of 39.0° C and a swollen and erythematous right foot. Physical examination reveals palpable femoral pulses but no palpable distal pulses. The plantar surface of the foot is painful on deep palpation, and an ulcer under the first metatarsal head shows a small amount of purulent drainage. Which of the following is the next step in this patient's management?

(A) Performance of an emergent lower extremity arteriogram
(B) Administration of oral antibiotics and close observation
(C) Administration of antibiotics and surgical wound débridement
(D) Emergent performance of a below-the-knee amputation
(E) Emergent performance of a guillotine amputation

17. A 65-year-old man with a history of hypertension presents to the emergency room 1 hour after acute onset of right arm and leg weakness and dysarthria. During evaluation, the patient is noted to have continued right arm and leg weakness. The patient was also still dysarthric. An immediate head computed tomography (CT) scan without contrast was performed and was read as "normal." Which of the following statements is true regarding this patient's condition?

(A) This patient's findings are most likely secondary to a transient ischemic attack
(B) This patient may have sustained rupture of an intracerebral arteriovenous malformation
(C) Heparin should not be administered given the potential for intracerebral hemorrhage
(D) A repeat CT scan may demonstrate the presence of an ischemic stroke
(E) Thrombolytic agents (e.g., tissue plasminogen activator) provide no benefit in the presence of a normal CT scan

18. A 55-year-old smoker presents to the office with a 2-day history of a worsening ulcer over the medial portion of her right ankle and pain in the extremity below the knee. She denies recent trauma to the area. On examination, the patient is noted to have a 3-cm ulcer over the medial portion of the right ankle. There is no purulence, but there is some oozing of dark blood. The distal right leg is noted to be pale. She is noted to have strong pulses over the right femoral artery although the leg is massively edematous. The right pedal pulse is slightly palpable but much weaker than the left pedal pulse. Which of the following is the most appropriate next step in the evaluation and management of this patient?

(A) An arteriogram should be performed immediately
(B) Doppler evaluation should be performed immediately
(C) The primary treatment is with intravenous (IV) antibiotic administration
(D) The primary treatment involves cessation of smoking
(E) An echocardiogram will most likely reveal the source of an embolus

Answers and Explanations

1-B. Prosthetic graft infection is a serious complication, with an associated mortality rate approaching 30%. This may frequently be related to disruption of the infected anastomosis site, leading to sudden severe arterial bleeding. The general approach for treating infected prosthetic grafts involves antibiotics, removing the entire prosthesis, and reestablishing vascular continuity through noncontaminated fields. Extra-anatomic routes of axillofemoral or femorofemoral grafts permit revascularization through a clean field distal to the original operative site. Antibiotics alone would be insufficient therapy in the presence of an infected graft. Revascularization with extra-anatomic bypass grafts helps prevent the need for amputation in an otherwise ischemic extremity.

2-E. Noninvasive vascular studies are an important complement to a detailed vascular history and physical examination. Sequential extremity pressure measurements allow determination of the ankle-brachial index (ABI) by dividing the ankle systolic blood pressure by the brachial pressure. Normally the ABI should be 1.0–1.1 in both extremities. In patients with intermittent claudication, the ABI is generally between 1.0 and 0.5, with an average value of 0.6, and in patients with more advanced ischemia, the ABI is generally less than 0.5. Arteriography and arterial duplex scanning are important diagnostic tests, but are not generally used for initial screening evaluation. The patient's clinical findings suggest intermittent claudication related to arterial insufficiency rather than venous disease, hence Doppler ultrasound is not useful.

3-B. The main concern in this situation is that ischemia of the colon may have developed as a result of interruption of flow to the inferior mesenteric artery without adequate collateral blood supply from the superior mesenteric or hypogastric arteries to the sigmoid colon. Diarrhea, especially if it is bloody, is one of the earliest manifestations of colonic ischemia. The incidence of ischemic colitis after aortic reconstruction is about 2%. Aortoenteric fistula is a late complication of aortic aneurysm repair, resulting from erosion of a false aneurysm at the proximal aortic suture line into the duodenum. Pseudomembranous colitis associated with antibiotic use typically occurs somewhat later in the postoperative course. The duodenum is well vascularized from several collateral sources and is at low risk of developing ischemia after abdominal aortic aneurysm repair. This patient is certainly at risk for stress gastritis, but the primary concern should be for the possibility of ischemic colitis.

4-D. When ischemic colitis is considered after aortic aneurysm repair, immediate proctosigmoidoscopy is important in the initial evaluation to assess colonic viability. Ischemic changes are visualized as pale patchy areas with membranes. Ischemic colitis may be limited to the mucosa or may be transmural. The adequacy of arterial flow and the viability of the colon can be evaluated intraoperatively by Doppler auscultation of the bowel mesentery, observation of bowel peristalsis, and measurement of the inferior mesenteric artery (IMA) stump pressure. A strong pulsatile Doppler signal in the mesentery, active sigmoid peristalsis, a chronically occluded IMA, or a patent IMA with stump pressure greater than 40 mm Hg predict viability of the colon postoperatively. However, none of these observations excludes the possibility of late sigmoid ischemia. Barium enema is not as accurate as sigmoidoscopy for determining the depth of injury and carries risks of contamination if perforation occurs.

5-C. Popliteal artery aneurysms are the most common arteriosclerotic peripheral aneurysm, and typically present in the seventh decade. Multiple aneurysms commonly accompany popliteal aneurysms; 50%–70% of patients have bilateral popliteal aneurysms, and abdominal aortic aneurysms (AAAs) are found in 70% of these patients. Once the diagnosis of a popliteal artery aneurysm is made, a search for associated, life-threatening aortic and other limb-threatening peripheral aneurysms must be undertaken. Angiography can be misleading in the diagnosis of aneurysms because of the presence of intraluminal thrombus. Once repair is planned, angiography is essential to define the patency of the distal vasculature. Early surgical treatment is recommended when a popliteal artery aneurysm is diagnosed because of the high incidence of complications. Thrombolytic therapy or thrombectomy before specific surgical treatment of a popliteal aneurysm is indicated in the presence of limb-threatening ischemia from thrombosis.

6-B. Asymptomatic carotid bruits occur in about 5% of the population over 50 years old. Unfortunately, carotid bruits do not always arise from significant carotid artery stenosis. Only 23% of patients identified to have bruits on physical examination have a significant carotid stenosis. The presence of a carotid bruit has little significance relative to the neurologic prognosis of the patient. Carotid bruit does, however, remain a significant predictor of symptomatic, life-threatening coronary artery disease. Despite the poor correlation between the presence of a carotid bruit and ipsilateral cerebral ischemia, bruits should not be ignored and should prompt a noninvasive evaluation to rule out significant carotid lesions.

7-E. Carotid color-flow duplex scanning uses real-time B-mode ultrasound and color-enhanced pulsed Doppler flow measurements to determine the extent of carotid stenosis with reliable sensitivity and specificity. It provides a rapid noninvasive method to quantify the degree of carotid stenosis and to assess morphologic characteristics. It is the single best screening test for evaluation of carotid disease and may be considered by some surgeons to be sufficient for planning operative intervention. Angiography remains the definitive method of evaluating carotid anatomy in most centers, but it is not advocated as a screening procedure because it is invasive and carries a small risk of neurologic complications. Aspirin may reduce the risk of stroke somewhat, but not as dramatically as carotid endarterectomy in patients with a high-grade stenosis. The role of warfarin in carotid occlusive disease remains controversial. An echocardiogram may be necessary later in the evaluation to rule out a cardiac source of emboli if a carotid source is not definitively identified. Stress thallium tests are used to identify patients who might benefit from coronary artery revascularization before undergoing aortic bypass grafting.

8-C. Carotid endarterectomy (CEA) is highly beneficial in patients with recent hemispheric or retinal transient ischemic attacks (TIAs) or nondisabling strokes and an ipsilateral high-grade carotid stenosis (70%–99%). The long-term risk of asymptomatic carotid stenosis is not fully defined. Patients with asymptomatic carotid artery disease contralateral to symptomatic lesions generally do not face an increased stroke risk without an antecedent TIA. About 10%–15% of these patients may develop TIAs related to the asymptomatic lesion, but less than 1% suffer a stroke without antecedent TIA. It appears that these patients with asymptomatic contralateral disease can be managed expectantly, and surgical intervention is indicated once the patient becomes symptomatic. Bilateral CEA is usually not performed because of risk of recurrent laryngeal nerve trauma, which, if bilateral, could result in a tracheostomy and because of the potential risk of bilateral strokes and subsequent death. Percutaneous transluminal angiography of the carotid artery is generally not considered safe for atherosclerotic lesions because of the risk of embolization during catheter manipulation and balloon inflation and deflation.

9-D. The collection of a cardiac arrhythmia, the sudden onset of severe abdominal pain, and gut evacuation strongly suggests acute embolic mesenteric ischemia. Abdominal pain out of proportion to findings on physical examination is characteristic of mesenteric ischemia. Diagnosis depends on clinical suspicion, followed by diagnostic angiography of the mesenteric vessels. Emboli tend to lodge at branch points of the superior mesenteric artery. After diagnosis, the patient is heparinized, volume-resuscitated, and taken emergently to the operating room for an embolectomy or vascular bypass to restore blood flow. Nasogastric decompression and bowel rest may be helpful in patients with a small bowel obstruction but not for suspected ischemia. Given this scenario, highly suggestive of mesenteric ischemia, performing a computed tomography (CT) scan, right upper quadrant (RUQ) ultrasound, or upper endoscopy to rule out other potential sources would unnecessarily delay the work-up.

10-B. All of the complications listed may occur after repair of an abdominal aortic aneurysm, particularly when dissection within the pelvis is required. With appropriate operative technique, most of them are uncommon except for changes in sexual function. Retrograde ejaculation has been reported in as many as two thirds of patients, and impotence in as many as one third of patients. These changes may result from injury to the autonomic nerve fibers overlying the anterior aorta near the origin of the inferior mesenteric artery, or injury to those fibers overlying the proximal left common iliac artery and aortic bifurcation. In addition, disturbance of pelvic blood flow during aortic reconstruction may result in impotence.

11-A. Long-term patency of lower extremity vein grafts is adversely affected by continued tobacco use, by poor-quality or small vein conduits, and by poor distal runoff. Patency rates achieved using prosthetic conduits in the lower extremities are generally lower than those achieved with autogenous veins, particularly with grafts terminating below the knee. Patency rates generally are higher when bypass is performed for claudication than for salvage of the limb because of the extent of the underlying pathologic process. Despite considerable controversy, there seems to be little difference in patency whether the reversed saphenous vein or in situ vein technique is used.

12-C. When an extremity has been subjected to ischemia and muscular necrosis occurs, reperfusion can result in metabolic acidosis and profound hyperkalemia. Rhabdomyolysis releases myoglobin, which precipitates in acid urine and produces renal tubular obstruction and renal failure. Myoglobinuria produces red urine that is free of red blood cells. Treatment requires assurance of an adequate volume status with administration of intravenous (IV) fluids, prompt reversal of hyperkalemia to prevent cardiac arrest (IV insulin and glucose), administration of sodium bicarbonate to alkalinize the urine and to treat the systemic metabolic acidosis, and possibly osmotic diuresis with mannitol to prevent renal tubular obstruction. Continuation of anticoagulation therapy is critical because the patient remains at significant risk of recurrent embolism. Renal arteriography is not initially indicated because arterial emboli rarely involve the renal vessels. Blood transfusion is not an immediate requirement in this setting.

13-A. The long-term patency rates of aortofemoral bypass grafts are reported to range from 70%–90%. Of those in which graft occlusion develops, the most common cause is progressive atherosclerosis, followed by anastomotic thrombosis. Anastomotic aneurysm is the second most common late complication of aortic graft insertion, seen in 3%–5% of patients, almost always at the femoral anastomosis. Graft infection and enteric fistula remain dreaded and difficult late problems but they are infrequent. Aortoenteric fistula should be a primary consideration in any patient with a previous abdominal aortic graft who has gastrointestinal bleeding; most often, bleeding is into the third portion of the duodenum from the proximal aortic suture line.

14-C. Associated coronary artery disease is the leading cause of late death after aortic reconstruction. Because atherosclerosis is a diffuse process, patients with signs or symptoms of occlusive peripheral vascular disease require thorough evaluation for associated coronary or cerebrovascular atherosclerosis. Aggressive preoperative use of stress thallium or dipyridamole thallium cardiac stress tests is justified in order to define a patient's operative risk and to identify patients who might benefit from coronary artery revascularization before undergoing aortic bypass grafting. Administration of beta-blockers may also help in the prevention of this complication in patients at risk. The other choices are all potential complications of aortic surgery but are not as prevalent as coronary artery disease.

15-D. Amaurosis fugax is characterized by ipsilateral blindness, described by the patient as being like a window shade being pulled down over the eye. It is a type of transient ischemic attack (TIA) and resolves completely within 24 hours of its onset. It is caused by emboli that travel through the ophthalmic artery, the first intracerebral branch of the internal carotid artery, and then obstruct the retinal artery. These emboli may be seen on funduscopic examination and are called Hollenhorst plaques. The facial, occipital, and posterior auricular arteries are branches of the external carotid artery. The vertebral arteries provide the posterior circulation to the brain.

16-C. Diabetic patients are particularly prone to foot and lower extremity infections as a result of a compromised immune system, associated vascular occlusive disease, and peripheral neuropathy. All infections in diabetic patients merit serious attention, and all patients with evidence of cellulitis or wet gangrene of either the digits, forefoot, or foot should be admitted. Wounds should be cultured, and empiric broad spectrum antibiotics effective against gram-negative, gram-positive, and anaerobic organisms should be initiated. Additionally, plain radiographs of the extremity should be obtained at the time of presentation to rule out gas in the soft tissue, osteomyelitis, fractures, and foreign bodies. Definitive management of the affected extremity depends on the extent of the infectious involvement, the presence of systemic signs, and the severity of the vascular occlusive disease. In the patient described, cellulitis, systemic signs, and wet gangrene mandate emergent operative débridement and open drainage. In the presence of extensive wet gangrene of the foot, a below-the-knee amputation or possibly a guillotine amputation through the distal tibia and fibula may be indicated. Lower extremity revascularization to salvage ischemic but viable tissue is frequently necessary for patients who present with wet gangrene.

17-D. Prompt early evaluation of patients with acute neurologic deficits is essential in the management of neurologic disorders such as intracerebral hemorrhage and ischemic stroke. A head computed tomography (CT) scan may not demonstrate acute ischemic changes until 6–8 hours after the onset of symptoms. Thus the absence of ischemic changes should not prevent initiation of treatment for a suspected stroke. The initial CT scan is generally performed to assess for the presence of intracerebral hemorrhage (i.e., rupture of arteriovenous malformation), which is usually easily identified even on an early CT scan. Early initiation of heparin is indicated in patients with acute stroke symptoms in the absence of intracerebral hemorrhage. In addition, it has recently been shown that thrombolytic agents such as tissue plasminogen activator may help improve outcome in patients with acute ischemic stroke if therapy can be initiated early (i.e., within 6 hours) in the presence of signs and symptoms suggestive of ischemia without intracerebral hemorrhage.

18-B. An awareness of other causes of extremity ulceration other than arterial insufficiency is necessary in the appropriate management of such patients. This patient has characteristic findings of a venous stasis ulcer, including the location over the medial malleolus, the presence of severe edema in the extremity, and venous oozing from the wound. Ulcers secondary to severe arterial insufficiency typically affect the distal portion of the toes initially although trauma to any portion of an ischemic extremity may result in ulcer formation. This patient's findings, in association with decreased unilateral distal pulses, suggests the presence of severe venous stasis secondary to venous obstruction (phlegmasia alba dolens). This may result from ileofemoral venous thrombosis leading to arterial vasospasm. This can be diagnosed by venous Doppler evaluation of the extremity. Intravenous antibiotics and smoking cessation may be beneficial, but the primary treatment involves administering heparin and thrombolytic agents to treat the thrombus formation. If severe ischemia is present, emergent surgical venous embolectomy is indicated.

2

Thoracic and Cardiac

Patrick E. Parrino

I. Diseases of the Chest Wall and Pleura

A. Chest wall neoplasms

1. **Types of chest wall tumors**
   —Fifty to sixty percent are primary.
   —The rest are metastatic.

2. **Benign tumors** of the **ribs** include
   —**osteochondromas (most common).**
   —chondromas.
   —fibrous dysplasia.
   —histiocytosis X.

3. **Primary malignant tumors** of the **chest wall**
   —are characterized in **Table 2-1.**

4. **Most tumors present**
   —as an **enlarging mass,** although pain may be present in 50%–60%.

5. **Preoperative evaluation**
   —should carefully look for malignancy elsewhere.
   a. **Radiography and computed tomography (CT)**
      —of the **chest** are used to characterize the lesion locally.
   b. An **abdominal CT scan**
      —helps to identify liver metastases and evaluate other potential primary tumors (e.g., renal cell carcinoma).
   c. **Biopsy**
      —may be indicated to assess the need for preoperative chemotherapy, radiation therapy, or both.

Table 2-1. Primary Malignant Tumors of the Chest Wall

Tumor	Presentation	Treatment
Chondrosarcoma (most common)	Solitary, slow growing, sometimes painful mass in patients older than 40 years	Complete resection with 4–5 cm margins; tends to recur locally
Plasmacytoma	Associated with systemic multiple myeloma; typically presents with pain in men 50–70 years	Systemic chemotherapy and local radiation therapy; surgery rarely indicated
Ewing sarcoma	Occurs in children with 2:1 male:female ratio; painful chest wall swelling with fever, fatigue, malaise, and weight loss	Combination of chemotherapy, surgery, and radiation therapy
Osteogenic sarcoma	Painful mass in children and young adults; vascular invasion and lung metastases are common	Combination of chemotherapy and wide surgical excision; no role for radiation therapy

B. Pleural effusions

—may be a sign of local or systemic disease.

1. Normally, **pleural fluid flows** from the parietal pleura into the pleural space (5–10 L/day).

—It is then **absorbed by the visceral pleura.**

2. **Pleural fluid may accumulate in the chest** if there is

—**increased hydrostatic pressure** on the visceral side [e.g., congestive heart failure (CHF)].

—**increased capillary permeability** (e.g., local inflammation from pneumonia).

—**decreased plasma colloid oncotic pressure** (e.g., hypoalbuminemia).

—**increased negative intrapleural pressure** (e.g., atelectasis causing failure of the lung to expand during inspiration).

—**impaired drainage of the pleural space** because of lymphatic obstruction.

3. **Characteristic symptoms**

—include **pleuritic chest pain and dyspnea.**

4. **Effusions** of 350–400 mL

—result in "blunting" of the costophrenic angle on chest radiograph.

5. **Biochemical and cytologic analysis**

—of pleural fluid may be of diagnostic value.

   a. **Pleural effusions are classified** as **transudates or exudates (see *BRS General Surgery,* Table 2-5).**

    b. Fifty to sixty percent of malignant pleural effusions may be diagnosed in this manner.

  6. Treatment

    a. Small pleural effusions

      —generally resolve with treatment of the underlying cause of the effusion.

    b. Larger non-neoplastic effusions

      —require only diagnostic thoracentesis or temporary **chest tube drainage.**

    c. Effusions caused by malignancy

      —within the mediastinum or obstruction of lymphatics by tumor may respond to chemotherapy or radiation therapy.

      —If the effusion is symptomatic, thoracentesis may provide palliation.

    d. For recurrent or refractory effusions

      —pleural drainage, **followed by chemical pleurodesis** may be necessary.

      —Chemical pleurodesis uses a sclerosing agent (e.g., tetracycline, talc) to produce inflammation and permanent apposition of the visceral and parietal pleura.

      —Operative mechanical pleurodesis is sometimes required and involves inducing abrasions on the pleural surface to produce inflammation.

C. Empyema

—is an accumulation of purulent material in the pleural space.

  1. Occurrence

    —Over 50% are **secondary to pneumonia.**

    —**Twenty-five percent occur as a result of complications** of esophageal, pulmonary, or mediastinal **surgery.**

  2. Empyemas may be

    —acute or chronic.

    —localized or diffuse.

  3. Presenting **symptoms** include

    —**pleuritic chest pain.**

    —**fever.**

    —heaviness or discomfort on the affected side.

    —productive cough.

    —shortness of breath.

  4. Chest radiography

    —may reveal a pneumonia with a large pleural effusion or opacification of one hemithorax.

    —A **chest CT may help differentiate empyema from a lung abscess.**

  5. Fluid obtained from thoracentesis should be examined for

—Gram stain.

—**culture and sensitivity.**

—**biochemical analysis.**

6. **Empyema fluid** will often have

—a white blood cell (WBC) count greater than 15,000 cells/μL.

—a protein level more than 2.5–3.0 mg/dL.

—a specific gravity higher than 1.018.

7. **Treatment** generally involves

—therapeutic thoracentesis **or chest tube drainage.**

—**intravenous (IV) antibiotics.**

—treatment of the cause of the empyema.

8. If **pleural scarring develops**

—that causes lung trapping and failure of expansion, decortication (surgical removal of the fibrous peel) may be necessary.

D. Spontaneous pneumothorax

—results from rupture of a **subpleural bleb** typically located in the **apex of the upper lobe** or the superior segment of the lower lobe.

1. **Occurrence**

—This may **occur in patients** with **severe emphysema.**

—It **also classically occurs in tall, healthy, young, asthenic males** with long, narrow chests.

2. The **right lung** is more commonly involved than the left.

3. **Most episodes occur** when the patient is sedentary, not active.

4. **Catamenial pneumothorax**

—occurs in temporal relation to **menstruation.**

—is caused by defects in the visceral pleura caused by **endometrial implants.**

5. **Patients present with**

—**chest pain and shortness of breath** (95%).

—cough (10%).

6. **Complications**

a. There is a **50% recurrence rate**

—after an initial spontaneous pneumothorax.

b. A **tension pneumothorax**

—occurs in 2%–3% of patients (see *BRS General Surgery,* Chapter 8 III B 1).

7. **Treatment**

a. **Asymptomatic patients**

—with minimal pleural air may be observed with frequent chest films.

—Air is absorbed from the pleural cavity at about 1% per day.

    b. Symptomatic patients

        —should be treated with an **apical chest tube.**

        —Ninety-five percent of patients will have resolution of the air leak within 12–24 hours.

    c. Indications for surgery include

        —recurrent **pneumothorax.**

        —**continued air leak** or failure of the lung to re-expand after 3–5 days of therapy with a functioning, well-positioned chest tube.

        —**massive air leak** with failure to re-expand the lung after 24 hours.

        —bilateral **pneumothoraces,** either simultaneous or at different times.

        —**occupations** for which a recurrent pneumothorax would constitute a **significant risk to life** (e.g., mountain climber, diver, airline pilot).

        —patients living in **remote areas.**

        —large **bullae.**

    d. Surgery

        —consists of **stapling apical blebs.**

        —**performing pleurodesis.**

E. Chylothorax

—results from **injury to the thoracic duct** with leakage of chyle into the pleural space.

1. Injuries below the T5–6 level

—usually result in a right-sided chylothorax, whereas injuries above this level result in left-sided chylous effusions.

2. Etiologies

—In **adults 50% are due to tumor,** with 75% of these due to lymphoma.

—Other etiologies include **traumatic or iatrogenic injury.**

3. Characteristics of pleural fluid obtained by thoracentesis include

—milky appearance of the pleural fluid.

—protein at 2.2–5.9 g of protein/100 mL (about 50% of plasma).

—a lymphocyte count of 400–6800/μL.

—a specific gravity of 1.012–1.025.

—significant staining of fat with Sudan red.

—a triglyceride level higher than 110 mL/dL.

—characteristic presence of chylomicra.

4. Treatment

    a. For **most chylothoraces** a trial of conservative therapy is indicated with

        —**chest tube drainage.**

        —**avoidance of enteral feeds with provision of total parenteral nutrition for nutritional support.**

—Some patients may respond well to institution of a low-fat, medium-chain triglyceride diet, which can also decrease chyle formation.

b. For massive or **persistent chyle leaks**

—**transthoracic ligation of the thoracic duct** is recommended.

F. Mesotheliomas

—are the most common primary tumor of the pleura.

1. There is a **relation between asbestos exposure** and the **development of mesothelioma.**

2. Mesotheliomas are divided into localized and diffuse types.

3. Localized

a. Benign mesotheliomas are

—usually pedunculated and asymptomatic.

—**treated by simple excision.**

b. Malignant mesotheliomas typically present with

—chest pain.

—cough.

—dyspnea.

—fever.

—**Treatment** is wide local excision.

4. Diffuse malignant mesothelioma

a. Extension into adjacent structures (chest, diaphragm) is common.

b. Nodal involvement and distant metastases (liver, lung, brain) are common.

c. Most common in patients 60–80 years old, but 25% of patients are under 50 with a male:female ratio of 2–5:1.

d. Usual **presenting symptoms** include **chest pain, dyspnea, cough,** and weight loss.

e. Useful **diagnostic tools** are CT scan, biopsy, and thoracentesis of pleural fluid.

f. Prognosis is generally dismal regardless of therapy (surgery, radiation therapy, or chemotherapy)

—Selected patients with stage I disease may benefit from excision including pneumonectomy.

II. Diseases of the Mediastinum

A. Mediastinitis

1. Etiologies

a. Acute mediastinitis

—is associated with a high mortality.

—most commonly results from **esophageal perforation.**

b. Other causes include

—sternotomy incision and infections spreading from the oropharynx.

2. **Air is frequently present in the mediastinum**

   —on chest radiograph or CT scan.

3. Mediastinitis occurring **after sternotomy** often presents with

   —**sternal instability.**

   —**fever.**

   —**purulent drainage from the wound.**

B. **Mediastinal tumors (Table 2-2)**

   1. **Most tumors of the mediastinum are asymptomatic**

      —but some patients will have symptoms including chest pain, cough, and dyspnea.

   2. Evidence of **invasion of adjacent structures**

      —[nerves, trachea, superior vena cava (SVC), chest wall] is **suggestive of malignancy.**

   3. **Diagnosis**

      a. **CT scan or magnetic resonance imaging** (MRI) is used to locate and characterize the mass.

      b. **CT-guided fine needle aspiration** or surgical biopsy may be diagnostic.

   4. **Treatment**

      a. **For most masses**

         —excisional biopsy is the treatment of choice.

Table 2-2. Tumors of the Mediastinum

Tumors	Characteristics
Anterior and Superior Mediastinum	
Thymoma	25% malignant, 75% will develop myasthenia gravis within 10 years
Teratoma	Composed of multiple embryonic germ cell layers; 10%–20% are malignant
Thyroid tumors or goiter	Related to abnormal migration of thyroid tissue
Lymphoma (often T cell)	Lymph node biopsy often diagnostic
Parathyroid tumors	10% of adenomas found here secondary to abnormal migration of parathyroid glands
Lymphangiomas, lipomas	Generally benign and asymptomatic
Middle Mediastinum	
Pericardial cysts	75% occur in right cardiophrenic angle
Bronchogenic cysts	Originates from primordial ventral foregut tissue; presents as smooth mass involving trachea or bronchi near carina
Posterior Mediastinum	
Neurogenic tumors (neurofibromas, ganglioneuromas)	Arise from neural crest tissue such as sympathetic nerve trunks; in adults most are benign; in children most are malignant
Enteric cysts	Originate from dorsal foregut; associated with esophagus; may contain gastric epithelium that can bleed or ulcerate

    b. Neurogenic tumors

      —are treated with resection; however, 10% may have intraspinal involvement requiring simultaneous spinal surgery.

    c. Teratomas

      —are generally treated with a **combination of chemotherapy and excision** using α-fetoprotein and carcinoembryonic antigen (CEA) as markers of adequate treatment.

    d. Thymomas

      —are treated with **excision** via a sternotomy with postoperative chemotherapy for malignant thymomas.

    e. Lymphomas

      —are generally treated with **chemoradiation therapy** alone and do not require surgery.

C. Superior vena cava syndrome

—results from **obstruction of the SVC.**

  1. Etiology

    a. The **most common cause**

      —is **right upper lobe bronchogenic carcinoma.**

    b. Other causes include **benign conditions** such as

      —granulomatous disease.

      —idiopathic mediastinal fibrosis.

      —goiter.

      —bronchogenic cysts.

  2. Signs and symptoms include

    —facial and upper extremity edema.

    —distension of the veins of the head, neck, arms, and upper thorax.

    —rubor of the upper half of the torso, arms, and head.

    —periorbital swelling.

    —a "full" feeling in the head.

    —roaring in the ears made worse by lying supine.

  3. Diagnosis

    —can be made using conventional angiography or MRI in conjunction with biopsy of causative lesions.

  4. Cure is usually not possible

    —because most patients have malignant disease that has extensively invaded the mediastinum.

  5. Radiation therapy, chemotherapy, or both; or venous bypass grafting can provide acute relief.

III. Diseases of the Trachea

  A. Tumors of the trachea

    1. Tracheal tumors are **quite rare** but may include

—squamous cell carcinoma.

—adenoid cystic carcinomas.

—carcinoid tumors.

2. **Manifestations** may include

—stridor.

—cough.

—hemoptysis.

—recurrent pneumonia.

3. **Treatment**

—**Surgical excision** is generally the treatment of choice.

B. **Tracheal stenosis**

—may result from **localized tracheal ischemia** secondary to prolonged intubation with cuffed endotracheal tubes.

1. **To avoid this type of stenosis**

—tubes with low pressure and high volume cuffs should be used.

2. **Flexible bronchoscopy**

—is diagnostic.

—may allow for débridement of obstructing granulation tissue.

C. **Tracheoinnominate artery fistula**

1. Although rare, this **may result from erosion of an endotracheal tube or tracheostomy tube into the innominate artery.**

2. **Acute severe hemorrhage from the endotracheal tube** is diagnostic.

3. **Treatment** involves **both**

—rapid overinflation of the cuff or digital compression through a tracheostomy.

—emergent resection of the affected segment of the innominate artery.

IV. Diseases of the Lung

A. **Anatomy**

1. There are 3 lobes of the right lung and 2 lobes of the left lung.

2. Each of the lobes is divided into functionally distinct segments with individual segmental bronchi, arteries, and veins.

B. **Benign lung lesions**

1. **Lung abscess**

—most commonly develops **after aspiration pneumonia.**

a. The **most common sites of aspiration** are

—the **posterior segment of the upper lobe.**

—the **superior segment of the lower lobe.**

b. Bronchoscopy

—may be used to **identify obstructing endobronchial masses** contributing to abscess formation.

c. Treatment

(1) **Antibiotic therapy** is used to cover aerobic and anaerobic bacteria.

(2) **Pulmonary physiotherapy** and postural drainage are also important.

(3) **Operative treatment is required in fewer than 10% of patients.**

—When indicated, pulmonary resection is the recommended procedure.

2. Benign tumors

a. Hamartomas

—are the most frequently occurring benign neoplasms.

(1) A hamartoma is an **unusual arrangement of normal cells.**

(2) **Cartilage** is the most frequent tissue involved in the lung.

(3) These often present as **slow growing, solitary nodules** that may have characteristic **"popcorn" calcification on radiograph or CT scan.**

(4) **If the lesion is clearly a hamartoma**

—**asymptomatic tumors** may be followed on serial chest radiographs.

—**symptomatic lesions** (e.g., cough, pain, shortness of breath) are generally **resected.**

b. Arteriovenous (AV) malformations

—result from direct connection between the pulmonary artery and vein.

(1) **AV malformation lesions**

—are frequently associated with Rendu-Osler-Weber disease (hereditary hemorrhagic telangiectasia).

—occur as pulmonary nodules.

(2) **Associated symptoms** include

—dyspnea.

—hemoptysis.

—embolic neurologic events.

(3) **Treatment** involves

—**emobolization therapy** using percutaneous catheters.

C. Malignant lung lesions

1. Incidence and risk factors

a. Lung cancer

—is the **second most common** malignancy in the United States.

—is the **leading cause of cancer death.**

b. The male:female ratio is 2:1.

c. Ninety percent of lung cancers are associated with smoking.

—**Patients who stop smoking reduce their risk of developing lung cancer,** but it may take as long as 15 years to reach the risk of the general population.

d. Other **risk factors** include

—environmental exposures, such as asbestos.

—second hand smoke.

2. Small cell lung cancers (SCCA)

—make up 20% of the lung cancers.

a. These cancers are **neuroendocrine** in origin.

b. The **classic SCCA** is **oat cell carcinoma** with small, round uniform cells.

c. These tumors are **usually disseminated at time of diagnosis;** thus, fewer than 10% of all SCCA patients are candidates for surgery.

d. Lesions often present as **asymptomatic nodules** seen on radiograph.

—Patients may, however, present with **cough, hemoptysis, pneumonia,** or **weight loss.**

e. CT scan characterizes the local extent of the lesion as well as spread of the tumor to the mediastinum or abdomen (e.g., adrenals, liver).

f. Patients with **small peripheral tumors** and no nodal involvement (T1–2N0) have a 50% five-year survival with resection.

g. Other lesions are **generally treated with chemotherapy; however, overall 5-year survival is only 10%.**

3. Non–small cell lung cancers (NSCCA)

—make up 80% of the lung cancers.

a. Only 30% of patients with NSCCA have potentially resectable tumors.

b. NSCCA are divided into **4 subgroups.**

(1) Squamous cell carcinomas

—generally present as **central lesions.**

(2) Adenocarcinomas

—generally present as a **peripheral lung lesions.**

—**Bronchoalveolar variants** of adenocarcinomas may be **multifocal.**

(3) Undifferentiated large cell carcinomas

—are the least common type.

(4) Mixed tumors

—are comprised of a combination of the tissue types.

c. Most lesions present as **asymptomatic nodules** on radiograph.

(1) Some may present, however, with hemoptysis, atelectasis, pneumonia, pain, or weight loss.

(2) Tumors in the apex of the lung may result in compression or invasion of

—the brachial plexus, causing pain or arm weakness,

—the sympathetic ganglia, causing ptosis, miosis, enophthalmos, and decreased facial sweat ipsilaterally **(Pancoast tumors).**

d. **Bronchoscopic or CT-guided needle biopsy** may be performed for centrally or peripherally located lesions, respectively.

e. **Preoperative staging** is essential for determining resectability **(Table 2-3).**

(1) Overall, **nodal status is the single most important predictor of survival.**

(2) The **most common sites of metastases** are
  —brain.
  —supraclavicular nodes.
  —contralateral lung.
  —bone.
  —liver.
  —adrenal glands.

(3) **Mediastinoscopy**
  —may be performed if there is radiographic evidence of mediastinal adenopathy (N2 or N3 disease).

f. **Operability must be determined** to see if the patient is able to tolerate surgery and the subsequent loss of functional lung parenchyma.

(1) Underlying **cardiac disease** should be identified.

Table 2-3. Tumor-Node-Metastasis (TNM) Staging System for Non-Small Cell Carcinoma of the Lung

Primary Tumor	
Tis	Carcinoma in situ
T1	Tumor $\leq$ 3 cm
T2	Tumor > 3 cm, tumor that invades visceral pleura
T3	Any size within 2 cm of carina, extension into chest wall, diaphragm, pericardium
T4	Any size with invasion of heart, great vessels, trachea, esophagus, vertebrae, or malignant pleural effusion

Nodal Involvement	
N0	No nodal involvement
N1	Peribronchial and/or ipsilateral hilar nodes
N2	Mediastinal or subcarinal nodes
N3	Scalene of supraclavicular nodes or contralateral nodes

Distant Metastasis	
M0	No distant metastasis
M1	Distant metastasis

Stage Grouping	
Stage I	T1N0M0, T2N0M0
Stage II	T1N1M0, T2N1M0
Stage III	N2 or N3 disease, any T3 or T4
Stage IV	M1 disease

        (2) If forced expiratory volume (FEV$_1$)

           —is **greater than 2.2 L, then the patient can generally tolerate lung resection.**

           —is **less than 0.8 L,** then the patient is **generally not operable.**

        (3) Hypercarbia

           —[partial pressure of carbon dioxide (pCO$_2$)] greater than 50 mm Hg, also connotes inoperability.

    g. Treatment

        (1) Stage I and II disease

           —**Surgical resection** is the treatment of choice in operable patients.

        (2) Stage IIIa

           —is usually treated with a combination of surgery, chemotherapy, and radiation therapy.

        (3) Surgery may involve

           —**resection of a lung segment, lobe,** or an **entire lung on one side (pneumonectomy).**

           —**sampling of enlarged or suspicious lymph nodes.**

        (4) Chemotherapy

           —has **not** been shown to affect overall mortality.

        (5) Radiation therapy

           —decreases local recurrence rates in stage II and III cancers but has not been shown to increase survival.

    h. Recurrent disease

      —most frequently presents as distant metastases rather than local recurrence.

        (1) Brain metastasis is most common.

        (2) As many as **80% of recurrences occur within the first 2 years** after surgery.

4. Solitary pulmonary nodule

    a. Many patients may present with an asymptomatic solitary pulmonary nodule ("coin lesion") found on a chest radiograph.

    b. Overall, **10% or less of these lesions are malignant.**

    c. These **lesions may represent**

      —primary lung carcinoma.

      —benign lung tumors.

      —AV fistula.

      —granulomatous disease (e.g., tuberculosis, histoplasmosis).

      —metastatic disease.

    d. The potential **risk for malignancy** is affected by many factors, including

      —**patient age.**

      —history (e.g., history of smoking, or of exposure to tuberculosis).

      —characteristics of the lesion on radiograph and CT scan.

—growth patterns of the lesion.

e. A simplified algorithm for evaluation

—of a patient with a solitary pulmonary nodule is depicted in **Figure 2.1.**

f. Biopsy of a solitary pulmonary nodule

—may be performed with bronchoscopy, thoracoscopy, or percutaneously in some patients with indeterminate lesions on radiograph.

5. Pulmonary metastases

a. Some patients with **isolated pulmonary metastases from other sites may benefit from wedge resection** of these lung lesions.

b. Lesions that may be amenable to resection of pulmonary metastases include

—colon cancer.

—renal cell carcinomas.

—melanoma.

—endometrial carcinoma.

V. Diseases of the Heart

A. Ischemic heart disease (IHD)

1. The **normal anatomy**

—of the coronary vessels on a coronary angiogram is depicted in **Figure 2.2.**

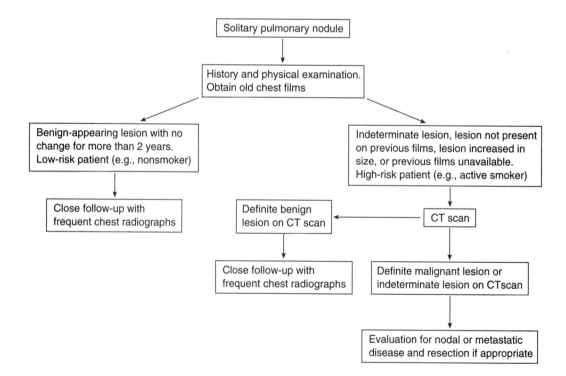

Figure 2.1. Evaluation of a solitary pulmonary nodule. CT = computed tomography.

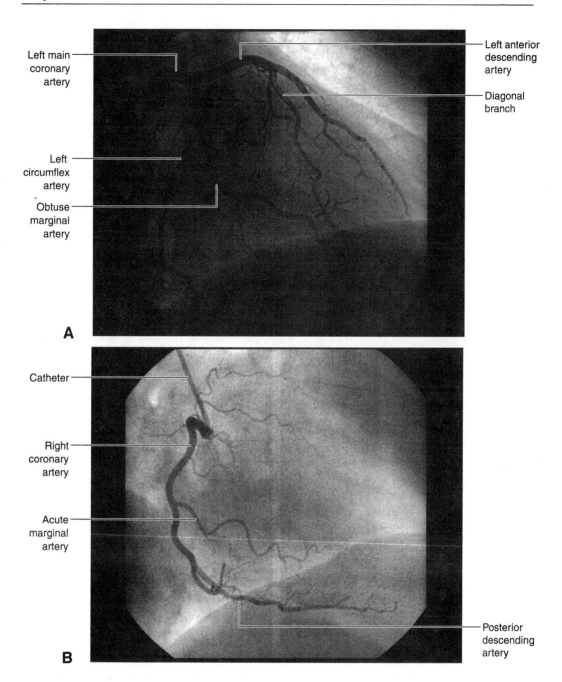

Figure 2.2. Normal coronary angiogram demonstrating the left (*A*) and right (*B*) coronary heart systems.

a. If the **posterior descending artery** arises

—from the **right** coronary vessels, these patients are considered **right dominant (90%).**

—from the **circumflex,** they are considered **left dominant.**

b. **Most atherosclerotic lesions**

—are located in the proximal portion of the vessels.

2. **Risk factors** for the development of IHD include

   —smoking.

   —hypertension.

   —male gender.

   —family history.

   —hyperlipidemia.

   —diabetes mellitus.

3. The **coronary veins have the lowest oxygen tension** of any tissue because of the high myocardial oxygen extraction rate (75%).

4. **Patients with IHD may present** with

   —stable or unstable angina.

   —myocardial infarction (MI).

   —arrhythmias.

   —sudden cardiac death (i.e., from ventricular fibrillation).

   —CHF.

5. **IHD is frequently managed medically** with a combination of

   —nitrates.

   —β blockers.

   —calcium channel blockers.

   —aspirin.

6. An **acute MI** may require additional therapy with **heparin and thrombolytic agents** such as tissue plasminogen activator (TPA) or **streptokinase.**

7. **Percutaneous transluminal angioplasty (PTCA)**

   —is frequently successful at dilating stenotic vessels.

   —is **used to treat most cases of severe IHD.**

8. **Coronary artery bypass grafting** (CABG)

   a. **Indications for CABG include**

      —**unstable angina** refractory to medical therapy with an inability to perform angioplasty or failed angioplasty.

      —significant **disease** of the **left main coronary artery.**

      —**three-vessel disease** with decreased left ventricular function.

      —**angina persisting** after an MI.

      —**anatomic complications** of disease (e.g., injured papillary muscle).

   b. **Relative contraindications to CABG** include

      —**diffuse distal coronary disease or poor ventricular function** (ejection fraction less than 20%) with refractory CHF.

   c. **During most cardiac surgeries, cardiopulmonary bypass** (CPB) is used to maintain tissue perfusion and provide **gas exchange** during circulatory arrest.

      (1) Blood is drained from the right atrium, passes through the CPB apparatus for gas exchange, and is infused directly into the aorta through catheters.

      (2) **Cardiac arrest** is maintained using coronary infusion of **high-**

potassium solutions (cardioplegia) in addition to maintaining **myocardial hypothermia** with cold solutions.

    d. **Vessels most commonly used for bypassing** diseased coronary segments include the **inferior mammary arteries (IMA) and saphenous vein grafts (SVG).**

    e. The **overall perioperative mortality** rate for CABG is **1%–2%.**
        —This rate may be as high as 10%–25% in the setting of an acute MI.

    f. Complications

        (1) **Immediate postoperative complications** may include
            —hypotension.
            —cardiac tamponade.
            —hemorrhage.
            —arrhythmias.

        (2) **Postpericardiotomy syndrome**
            —is a noninfectious pericarditis that presents within a few weeks of surgery.

            (a) **Signs and symptoms** include
                —fever.
                —chest pain.
                —dyspnea.
                —pericardial friction rub with ST segment elevation in multiple leads.

            (b) **Treatment**
                —involves administration of nonsteroidal anti-inflammatory drugs (NSAIDs).

        (3) **Recurrence**
            (a) **Early recurrence:** (less than 5 years) of angina secondary to progressive atherosclerosis in the native coronary arteries.
            (b) **Late recurrence:** (more than 7 years) secondary to atherosclerosis in the grafts.

        (4) **Sternal wound infection** and sternal dehiscence.

  9. **Surgery for complications of IHD**

    a. **Left ventricular aneurysms**
      —may occur in 5%–15% of patients after a large transmural MI.

        (1) **Presentation** may include
            —CHF.
            —arrhythmias.
            —angina.

        (2) **Indications for surgical repair** include
            —**refractory symptoms or arrhythmias.**
            —**large aneurysms** (larger than 5 cm).

    b. **Acute ventricular septal defect (VSD)**
      —**classically occurs 5–7 days after an MI.**
      —presents with acute CHF and a harsh pansystolic murmur.

        (1) **Diagnosis** is supported by a **step-up in oxygen saturation** (over 10%) between the left atrium and pulmonary artery **secondary to left-to-right shunting.**

(2) Surgical repair with placement of a patch over the defect is definitive therapy.

c. **Acute mitral regurgitation**

—**results from injury to the papillary muscles.**

—may be associated with a very high mortality.

—characteristically presents with acute **CHF and a holosystolic murmur** radiating to the axilla after an MI.

(1) Initial **medical therapy** is focused on afterload reduction (e.g., nitroprusside).

(2) Surgery involves repair of the papillary muscle and CABG to affected territory.

B. **Acquired valvular heart disease**

1. **Patients can be classified** based upon the severity of their symptoms related to cardiac disease using the New York Heart Association (NYHA) classification system **(Table 2-4).**

2. **Aortic stenosis (AS) [Table 2-5]**

—**causes early left ventricular hypertrophy.**

—is generally treated by replacing the native valve with a mechanical or biological prosthetic device.

3. Persistent **aortic regurgitation (AR)** [see Table 2-5]

—may result in eventual left ventricular dilation and subsequent hypertrophy.

—is also treated with valve replacement.

4. **Mitral regurgitation (MR)** [see Table 2-5]

—may lead to left atrial enlargement and eventual left ventricular failure.

a. Surgical options include **replacing the mitral valve or repairing the mitral valve via an annuloplasty.**

b. Injured papillary muscles resulting in MR may also be repaired or reimplanted.

5. **Mitral stenosis (MS)** [see Table 2-5]

—may lead **to early left atrial enlargement and pulmonary hypertension.**

a. **Division of the fused valves (commissurotomy)** is the initial surgical therapy.

Table 2-4. New York Heart Association (NYHA) Classification of Severity of Heart Disease

Class	Symptoms
Class I	No symptoms
Class II	Chest pain or dyspnea with heavy exertion
Class III	Chest pain or dyspnea with mild exertion
Class IV	Chest pain or dyspnea at rest

Table 2-5. Acquired Valvular Heart Disease

Lesion	Cause	Presentation	Indications for Surgery
Aortic stenosis (AS) [most common]	Calcification of bicuspid valve, rheumatic heart disease, senile calcification or normal aortic valve	Angina→syncope →CHF (bad prognosis); sudden cardiac death from ventricular fibrillation; patients with bicuspid valves present between age 40–60, while others present between 60–80 years of age	Symptomatic disease, aortic outflow surface area < 0.5 cm^2; pressure gradient across valve > 50 mm Hg
Aortic regurgitation (AR)	Myxomatous degeneration (Marfan's), rheumatic heart disease, calcification, endocarditis, aortic dissection with dilation of aortic root	Arrhythmias, angina, CHF, widened pulse pressure, rapid onset CHF if acute AR caused by aortic dissection	Acute severe disease, NYHA III or IV, AR refractory to medical therapy, worsening LV function
Mitral regurgitation (MR)	Rheumatic heart disease, calcification, severe mitral valve prolapse, endocarditis, papillary muscle injury after MI	Arrhythmias (atrial fibrillation), eventual CHF, systemic embolization from left atrial enlargement and thrombus formation (rare)	Acute onset MR from papillary muscle injury, NYHA III or IV, progressive refractory MR
Mitral stenosis (MS)	Rheumatic heart disease 20–30 years after rheumatic fever	Arrhythmias (atrial fibrillation), CHF, hemoptysis from chronic pulmonary hypertension, systemic embolization	NYHA III or IV, mitral valve area < 1 cm^2, symptomatic disease refractory to medical therapy, pressure gradient across valve > 10 mm Hg
Tricuspid regurgitation (TR) and tricuspid stenosis (TS)	Right ventricular hypertrophy (most common cause of TR), endocarditis from IV drug abuse, rheumatic heart disease	Right-sided heart failure: hepatomegaly, peripheral edema, jugular venous distension, ascites	Surgery rarely necessary; resulting right-sided heart failure, pressure gradient across valve > 4 mm Hg

CHF = congestive heart failure; IV = intravenous; NYHA = New York Heart Association functional classification system for heart disease; LV = left ventricle; MI = myocardial infarction.

    b. Mitral valve replacement may rarely be required for recurrent disease.

  6. Tricuspid regurgitation (TR) [see Table 2-5]

      —is most commonly caused by right ventricular dilation resulting from left-sided heart failure and pulmonary hypertension.

      —Isolated tricuspid valve disease from endocarditis may be treated with valve excision in the absence of pulmonary hypertension or valve replacement.

7. Tricuspid stenosis (TS) [see Table 2-5]

—secondary to rheumatic heart disease may be repaired **with valve re**placement or commissurotomy.

8. Considerations in heart valve replacement

a. Valvular replacement

—can be performed with **mechanical or biological valves.**

b. Examples of **mechanical valves** include

—the St. Jude's bileaflet hinged valve and the Starr-Edwards **caged ball valves.**

(1) These valves require **life-long anticoagulation therapy,** [e.g., coumarin (Coumadin)] because of the **high risk of valvular thrombus** formation and subsequent embolization.

(2) The risk of cerebral thromboembolization with these valves is 1%–5% a year despite anticoagulation, although this rate is variable.

(3) The **advantage of these valves is their durability.**

(4) Contraindications to chronic anticoagulation, and thus mechanical valve insertion include

—major **bleeding diathesis.**

—**noncompliant patient.**

—**patients at high risk for hemorrhagic stroke.**

—**current or planned pregnancy.**

(5) The normal locations of an aortic and mitral mechanical valve on chest radiograph are demonstrated in **Figure 2.3.**

c. The **most common type of xenograft,** or **biological valve, is the porcine valve,** although homografts (human cadaver valves) and bovine valves are also used.

(1) The **main disadvantage of tissue valves is their poor durability.**

—Fifty percent of valves require replacement within 13 years.

(2) Unlike mechanical valves, these do not require long-term anticoagulation, although brief postoperative anticoagulation (3–8 weeks) may be given.

(3) Because of rapid calcification of tissue valves in younger patients, use of these valves is relatively contraindicated in children and young adults.

(4) Chronic renal dialysis is also a contraindication to insertion of a tissue valve because of the propensity for rapid calcification of the valve.

C. Congenital heart disease

1. The 3 **most common congenital heart defects, respectively, are**

—**VSD.**

—**atrial septal defect (ASD).**

—**patent ductus arteriosus (PDA).**

2. Characteristics of many congenital heart defects

—are outlined in **Table 2-6.**

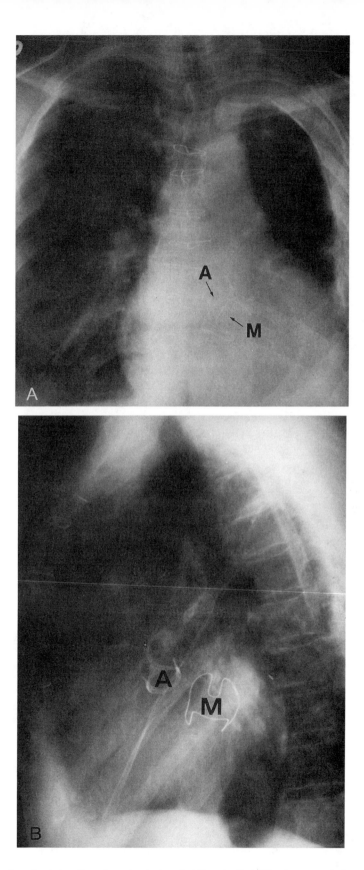

Figure 2.3. Normal anatomic location of mechanical aortic (A) and mitral (M) valves on anterior-posterior and lateral chest radiographs. (*A*) anterior-posterior view. (*B*) lateral view. (Reprinted with permission from Daffner RH: Pulmonary Imaging. In *Clinical Radiology: The Essentials,* 2nd ed. Edited by Daffner RH. Baltimore, Lippincott Williams & Wilkins, 1999, p 163.)

Table 2-6. Congenital Heart Defects

Defect	Pathophysiology	Features	Surgical Indications	Procedure
Ventricular septal defect (VSD)	L-to-R shunt through membranous (80%) or muscular septum	Early pulmonary hypertension, CHF, endocarditis; associated with other defects (e.g., PDA)	CHF, progressive pulmonary hypertension, large shunt ($Q_p/Q_s > 2.0$)	Spontaneous closure often occurs (25%–50%); patch closure of large defects after age 1
Atrial septal defect (ASD)	L-to-R shunt through ostium primum or secundum (80%)	Late onset pulmonary hypertension and CHF	Large shunt ($Q_p/Q_s > 2.0$)	Primary or patch closure of defect
Patent ductus arteriosus (PDA)	L-to-R shunt; failure of neonatal closure of ductus	Pulmonary hypertension, CHF, endocarditis	Urgent surgery for CHF, failed closure with indomethacin	Ligation or clipping of PDA at 1–2 years of age
Tetralogy of Fallot	R-to-L shunt; RV outflow obstruction, VSD, overriding aorta, RV hypertrophy	Cyanotic ("tet") spells relieved by squatting; boot-shaped heart on radiograph	Formal repair may be preceded by palliative subclavian artery to pulmonary artery (Blalock-Taussig) shunt	Correction of pulmonary outflow obstruction and VSD closure
Aortic coarctation	Narrowing of aorta near ligamentum arteriosum distal to left subclavian artery	Severe CHF with absent distal pulses, upper extremity hypertension in adults	Depends on age at presentation	Resection and reanastomosis, patch or flap aortoplasty
Transposition of the great vessels	R-to-L shunt; aorta originates from RV and pulmonary artery originates from LV	Causes cyanosis and CHF in newborns	Formal repair preceded by palliative balloon atrial septostomy (dilation of ASD)	Atrial or arterial switch procedure

L = left; R = right; CHF = congestive heart failure; RV = right ventricle; LV = left ventricle.

3. **Defects associated** with

—**left-to-right shunts** include ASD, VSD, and PDA.

—**right-to-left shunts** include tetralogy of Fallot and transposition of the great vessel.

4. In general, **lesions associated** with
   a. **left-to-right shunts present with CHF.**
      —In infants, CHF manifests as failure to thrive, tachycardia, tachypnea, and hepatomegaly.
   b. **right-to-left shunts present with cyanosis.**
      —Cyanotic heart disease may lead to polycythemia, strokes, brain abscesses, endocarditis, and hypertrophic osteoarthropathy (clubbing).

5. **Left-to-right shunts**

   —**characteristically cause pulmonary hypertension.**
   a. **Severe pulmonary hypertension**
      —resulting from a left-to-right shunt (e.g., VSD) may eventually cause **reversal of flow to a right-to-left shunt.**
      —This condition is known as **Eisenmenger syndrome.**
   b. **Prevention is crucial because this syndrome is generally considered irreversible** and is associated with a very high mortality.

D. **Cardiovascular support devices**

1. **Intra-aortic balloon pumps (IABP)**

   —may be used in some patients with hypotension caused by poor ventricular function.
   a. **Indications for IABP** include
      —refractory left ventricular failure after CPB.
      —refractory unstable angina.
      —being a bridge to surgery in patients with severe CHF.
   b. The **tip of the IABP catheter**
      —is placed in the descending thoracic aorta via the femoral artery.
   c. The **balloon is synchronized** with the patient's rhythm
      —to **inflate during diastole, causing increased aortic pressure and coronary flow.**
      —to **deflate during systole, causing a reduction in afterload** and cardiac demand.
   d. **IABP may exacerbate aortic regurgitation** and is therefore contraindicated in this setting.
   e. **Complications** include
      —lower extremity ischemia.
      —thromboembolic disease.
      —mesenteric ischemia.
      —renal failure.
      —paraplegia.

2. **Left ventricular assist device (LVAD)**

   a. **A LVAD may be used** in the setting of severe left-sided heart failure as a bridge to transplantation.

   b. **This device** drains blood from the left atrium or ventricle via cannulas.

      —It then pumps the blood back into the ascending aorta to bypass left ventricular function.

E. **Cardiac tumors**

   1. The **most common malignancies of the heart** are **metastatic lesions.**

      a. **Metastatic lesions** include

         —carcinomas of the lung and breast.

         —melanoma.

         —lymphoma.

      b. Although rare, **primary sarcomas** and melanomas of the heart may occur.

   2. The **most common primary cardiac tumor** is a **benign myxoma.**

      a. These lesions **most commonly occur** in the **left atrium.**

      b. **Atrial myxomas** are generally pedunculated lesions that may lead to atrial **outflow obstruction or thromboembolic events.**

VI. Diseases of the Thoracic Aorta

A. **Aortic dissection**

   1. **Degeneration of the elastic fibers in the media** may result in

      —intimal tears.

      —**dissection of blood between the intimal and medial layers** of the aorta.

      —This degeneration is frequently referred to as cystic medial necrosis.

   2. **Risk factors**

      a. The **most common risk factor**

         —for aortic dissection is hypertension.

      b. **Other risk factors** include

         —myxomatous degeneration (Marfan's).

         —atherosclerosis.

         —aortic coarctation.

         —trauma.

         —infection (e.g., syphilis).

   3. **Types of dissections (Figure 2.4)**

      a. **Type A dissections**

         —involve the **ascending aorta** with or without the transverse or descending aorta.

      b. **Type B dissections**

         —**involve the descending aorta only.**

         —may also involve the renal or visceral vessels.

   4. **Presentation**

      a. **Characteristic symptoms** include

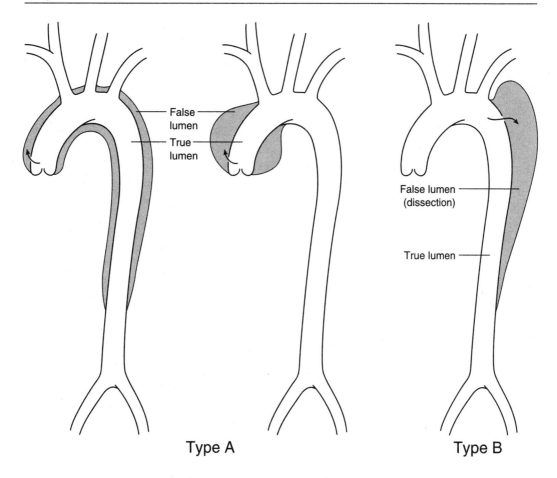

Figure 2.4. Type A and type B aortic dissections.

—acute onset of "tearing" chest pain with radiation to the back between the scapulae.

b. **Dissection mimics an acute MI,** which must be considered during evaluation.

c. **Blood pressures and pulses** may be asymmetrical in the upper extremities.

d. **Dissection can lead to**
   —cardiac tamponade.
   —acute aortic regurgitation.
   —hypotension secondary to rupture.

e. Patients generally have a **normal chest radiograph,** although a widened mediastinum may be noted in some cases.

5. **Diagnostic studies** may include

   —**CT scan with contrast.**

   —MRI.

   —an aortogram.

   —transesophageal echocardiogram in addition to evaluation of a potential MI.

6. **Treatment**
   a. **Type A dissections**
      —are generally repaired with **tube graft placement** with aortic valve replacement or repair if the aortic valve is involved (Bentall procedure).
   b. **Uncomplicated Type B dissections**
      —may be treated with **close monitoring and aggressive antihypertensive therapy** (e.g., nitroprusside, esmolol).
   c. **Complicated Type B dissections**
      —(e.g., persistent pain, progressive dissection) or sustained refractory hypertension **require surgical repair.**

B. **Aneurysms of the thoracoabdominal aorta** (see Chapter 1)

Review Test

Directions: Each of the numbered items or incomplete statements in this section is followed by answers or by completions of the statement. Select the ONE lettered answer or completion that is BEST in each case.

1. A 65-year-old man with a history of poorly controlled hypertension, diabetes, and gout presents to the emergency room with a 1-hour history of severe, sharp chest pain over the left sternal border in addition to severe pain in his back between the scapulae. He states that he was working in the yard when the pain developed. Chest radiograph shows no abnormalities and electrocardiogram demonstrates no ST changes. Administration of sublingual nitrates, intravenous morphine, and oxygen provide minimal relief of the chest and back pain. Which of the following is the most appropriate next step in the management of this patient?

(A) Immediate cardiac catheterization
(B) Administration of tissue plasminogen activator
(C) Aggressive fluid administration
(D) Performance of a chest computed tomography (CT) scan
(E) Continued observation

2. A 46-year-old, otherwise healthy woman presents to the office with complaints of a 3–4 month history of dyspnea on exertion and intermittent chest pain. She states that she has been experiencing lightheadedness particularly when she works in the yard and has had one episode where she almost fainted. During physical examination, she is noted to have a crescendo-decrescendo systolic murmur over the second right intercostal space radiating into the carotids and a narrow pulse pressure. Which of the following is the most likely primary etiology of this patient's disease?

(A) Calcification of a bicuspid valve
(B) Senile calcification of a normal valve
(C) Myxomatous valvular degeneration
(D) Bacterial endocarditis
(E) Aortic dissection and annular dilation

3. A 65-year-old man with no previous history of cardiopulmonary disease presents to the office for routine examination. Physical examination reveals a systolic murmur noted just to the right of the sternum in the second intercostal space that was not noted previously. Subsequent echocardiogram reveals aortic stenosis. Which of the following symptoms would predict the worst prognosis for this patient?

(A) Angina with vigorous exertion
(B) Syncopal episodes
(C) Frequent palpitations
(D) Angina with mild exertion
(E) Dyspnea at rest

4. A 54-year-old man presented to the emergency room with acute onset severe substernal chest pain and was found to have a progressing myocardial infarction (MI). The patient underwent successful angioplasty and despite having sustained a moderately sized anteroseptal MI, recovered well. Before discharge on hospital day 7, the patient acutely developed severe shortness of breath and tachypnea. Physical examination revealed a harsh pansystolic murmur. A pulmonary artery catheter was placed and demonstrated a right atrial partial pressure of oxygen (PO_2) of 60 and a PO_2 of 85 in the pulmonary trunk on 50% fraction of inspired oxygen (FIO_2). Which of the following is the most appropriate next step in the management of this patient?

(A) Surgical repair of the ventricular septum
(B) Repeat angioplasty of diseased vessel
(C) Ventilation-perfusion (V/Q) scan and heparin administration
(D) Coronary artery bypass grafting (CABG) of diseased vessel
(E) Pulmonary arteriogram and heparin administration

5. A 65-year-old man with a history of chronic obstructive pulmonary disease (COPD) and hypertension is found to have a suspicious lung nodule in the right upper lobe on chest radiograph performed for nonspecific respiratory complaints. A needle biopsy performed before referral to your clinic revealed a squamous cell carcinoma of the lung. Which of the following factors indicates that this patient should undergo surgical resection of this lesion?

(A) A 3-cm tumor involving segmental bronchi with a forced expiratory volume (FEV_1) of 0.8
(B) A 3-cm tumor involving segmental bronchi with positive ipsilateral hilar nodes and an FEV_1 of 1.9
(C) A 2-cm peripheral tumor without positive nodes with a resting partial pressure of carbon dioxide (PCO_2) of 59
(D) A 2-cm peripheral tumor with positive contralateral hilar nodes and a resting PCO_2 of 45
(E) A 1-cm peripheral tumor initially diagnosed on cytology of a small pleural effusion with an FEV_1 of 2.4

6. A 55-year-old man with a history of hypertension and chronic obstructive pulmonary disease (COPD) from chronic smoking is found to have a 4-cm nodule in the left upper lung lobe on radiography. Subsequent biopsies demonstrate characteristic oat cell carcinoma. Chest computed tomography (CT) and physical examination reveal enlarged lymph nodes in the mediastinum but not on the contralateral side. Supraclavicular nodes were also noted **not** to be enlarged. Which of the following is the most appropriate management strategy in this patient?

(A) Left upper lobectomy with postoperative mediastinal radiation therapy
(B) Left upper lobectomy with postoperative chemotherapy
(C) Administration of systemic chemotherapy alone
(D) Radiation therapy to the lesion and mediastinum alone
(E) Left upper lobectomy with resection of involved nodes

7. A 47-year-old man presents to the office with complaints of a persistent cough for 2–3 months. He is otherwise healthy and quit smoking about 20 years ago. On chest radiograph, he is found to have a solitary lung mass in the right middle lobe. A subsequent chest computed tomography (CT) scan reveals a 2-cm mass in the right middle lobe with characteristic popcorn calcifications consistent with a hamartoma. Which of the following would be the most appropriate management strategy in this patient if biopsy reveals a hamartoma?

(A) Performance of a right middle lobectomy
(B) Performance of a right pneumonectomy
(C) Observation with serial chest radiographs
(D) Wedge resection of the hamartoma
(E) Bronchoscopic resection of the hamartoma

8. A 64-year-old man presents to the emergency room with complaints of fever, cough, and right-sided chest pain. Chest radiograph reveals consolidation of the right lower lobe of the lung. Review of the patient's records reveals 2 previous episodes of pneumonia involving the right lower lobe in the past 4 months. Subsequent computed tomography (CT) scan reveals a 3-cm lung abscess. In addition to administering intravenous (IV) antibiotics, which of the following is the most appropriate management strategy for this patient?

(A) Chest physiotherapy
(B) Right lower lobectomy
(C) Wedge resection of abscess
(D) Surgical drainage of abscess
(E) Bronchoscopy

9. A 37-year-old woman presents to the office with complaints of fatigue and weight loss. Chest radiography reveals widening of the mediastinum, while abdominal computed tomography (CT) scan reveals enlargement of periaortic lymph nodes. Biopsy of the mediastinal mass reveals a lymphoma. Which of the following is the most appropriate therapy for this patient?

(A) Surgical resection of the mediastinal mass
(B) Mediastinal radiation therapy and chemotherapy
(C) Surgical resection of the mass and chemotherapy
(D) Mediastinal radiation therapy alone
(E) Surgical resection of the mass and retroperitoneal radiation therapy

10. A 42-year-old woman presents to the office with progressive profound muscle weakness and fatigue. Thorough evaluation reveals a diagnosis of myasthenia gravis. When discussing this disease with the patient, which of the following is an appropriate statement regarding this disease process?

(A) Symptoms of disease are related to an anti-acetylcholine antibody
(B) Over 90% of patients with myasthenia gravis will have a thymoma
(C) Over 90% of patients with a thymoma have myasthenia gravis
(D) Resection of a thymoma may relieve symptoms of myasthenia gravis
(E) In the absence of myasthenia gravis, thymomas do not require resection

11. A 35-year-old woman presents to the office with complaints of dyspnea on mild exertion and exercise intolerance. Chest radiograph reveals a mass in the anterior mediastinum. Biopsy of the mass reveals thyroid tissue with a diffuse lymphocytic infiltrate surrounding germinal centers. The patient is noted to have a decreased triiodothyronine (T_3) and thyroxine (T_4) and an elevated thyroid-stimulating hormone. Which of the following is the most likely diagnosis in this patient?

(A) Thyroid goiter with abnormal embryonic thyroid migration
(B) Locally invasive follicular cell carcinoma of the thyroid
(C) Locally invasive papillary carcinoma of the thyroid gland
(D) Mediastinal extension of a primary lymphoma
(E) Primary lymphoma of an ectopic thyroid gland

12. A 32-year-old, tall man presents to the emergency room with the complaint of acute onset sharp chest pain on the left. Chest film reveals a 30% pneumothorax on the left with no mediastinal shift and also reveals a large apical bleb in the left upper lobe. The patient's heart rate is 95 beats/min with a blood pressure of 125/78 mm Hg. The patient states that he is an airline pilot and also denies having any such previous episodes. Which of the following is the most appropriate management strategy in this patient?

(A) Chest tube thoracostomy and elective wedge resection of the bleb
(B) Chest tube thoracostomy alone
(C) Chest tube thoracostomy and left upper lobectomy
(D) Chest tube thoracostomy and pleurodesis
(E) Chest tube thoracostomy, wedge resection of the bleb, and pleurodesis

13. A 64-year-old man undergoes elective esophagectomy for Stage I esophageal carcinoma. On postoperative day 3, the patient develops consolidation of the right middle lung lobe associated with a worsening pleural effusion. Despite improvement of the pneumonia in the middle lobe with intravenous (IV) antibiotic administration, the effusion slightly increases in size. Which of the following is consistent with the diagnosis of an empyema?

(A) Strongly positive Sudan red staining
(B) Presence of chylomicra
(C) Red blood cells over 50,000/mL
(D) White blood cell count = 20,000 with 70% polymorphonuclear leukocytes
(E) Specific gravity of 1.014

14. A 67-year-old man with chronic obstructive pulmonary disease (COPD) and hypertension presents to the office with a 3–4 month history of worsening persistent cough. He has smoked 2 packs per day for 25 years. Chest radiograph reveals a 3-cm peripheral lung nodule in the apical region of the right upper lobe in addition to a right pleural effusion. Which of the following is the most appropriate next step in the evaluation of this patient?

(A) Bronchoscopic biopsy of the nodule
(B) Computed tomography (CT)-guided biopsy of the nodule
(C) Thoracentesis and pleural cytologic analysis
(D) Mediastinoscopy and biopsy of enlarged nodes
(E) No biopsy and performance of a right upper lobectomy

15. A 35-year-old woman presents to the office with complaints of worsening dyspnea on exertion. Subsequent evaluation reveals severe aortic stenosis with an aortic valve area of 0.4 cm^2 associated with left ventricular hypertrophy. Which of the following is an appropriate statement regarding the choice of valves used for replacement of the aortic valve?

(A) A porcine valve is favored over a mechanical valve because of the patient's life expectancy and the increased durability of the porcine valve

(B) A mechanical valve is favored over a porcine valve because of the lack of requirement of chronic anticoagulation with mechanical valves

(C) A mechanical valve is favored over a porcine valve because of the lack of requirement of immunosuppressive therapy for mechanical valves

(D) A mechanical valve is favored over a porcine valve because of the patient's life expectancy and the increased durability of the mechanical valve

(E) A porcine valve is favored over a mechanical valve because porcine valves perform better than mechanical valves when used specifically for aortic valve replacement

Answers and Explanations

1-D. This patient has the classic presentation of an aortic dissection with refractory chest pain in association with severe back pain between the scapulae. Aortic dissection frequently mimics acute myocardial infarction (MI) and thorough evaluation for potential myocardial ischemia should be performed. In addition, dissections of the ascending aorta may progress to dissection of the coronary vessels, causing acute myocardial ischemia. Although cardiac catheterization and administration of tissue plasminogen activator may be appropriate in the setting of an acute MI, the lack of definitive findings of myocardial ischemia and refractory chest and back pain should prompt evaluation of a possible dissection with a chest computed tomography (CT) scan. Observation alone would be inappropriate. Dissections are often associated with hypertension except in the setting of rupture, and blood pressure control (e.g., nitroprusside) rather than fluid administration would be appropriate therapies once the diagnosis is confirmed.

2-A. The most common causes of aortic stenosis include rheumatic heart disease that follows an episode of rheumatic fever by 20–30 years; calcification of a bicuspid valve, which typically occurs in patients 40–60 years old; and senile calcification of a normal aortic valve, which typically occurs in patients 60–80 years old. Myxomatous degeneration associated with Marfan's syndrome is an uncommon cause of aortic valve disease. Bacterial endocarditis is also an uncommon cause of aortic valve disease except in immunocompromised patients. Aortic dissection may rarely cause aortic regurgitation, not stenosis.

3-E. The symptoms associated with aortic stenosis have distinct prognostic value. In terms of progression of symptoms, angina generally precedes syncope, which precedes the development of congestive heart failure (CHF) and associated dyspnea with exertion or at rest. The overall life expectancy of untreated aortic stenosis presenting with angina is 3–5 years. For patients presenting with syncope the average is 2–3 years, while patients presenting with CHF have a life expectancy of 1–2 years. Palpations may be a consequence of either ischemia (e.g., angina) or CHF.

4-A. This is a classic presentation of a rupture intraventricular septum after an acute myocardial infarction (MI). Rupture typically occurs 5–7 days after the initial infarction. The oxygen differential between the right atrium and pulmonary trunk is characteristic of a ventricular septal defect (VSD) secondary to left-to-right shunting. Surgical repair with patching of the VSD is the definitive treatment. Repeat angioplasty or coronary artery bypass grafting (CABG) would not treat the VSD. A ventilation-perfusion (V/Q) scan and a pulmonary arteriogram would be helpful in the setting of a suspected pulmonary embolus but would not be appropriate in this setting.

5-B. There are several factors that determine resectability and operability of squamous cell carcinoma of the lung. A 3-cm tumor with positive ipsilateral hilar nodes is a stage II tumor (T2N1M0), which is considered a resectable lesion. However, patients with a forced expiratory volume (FEV_1) of 0.8 or less are considered inoperable because they are unlikely able to tolerate loss of lung parenchyma. In addition, a partial pressure of carbon dioxide (PCO_2) of 50 mm Hg or higher is also considered a criterion for inoperability. Positive contralateral hilar nodes are a stage III tumor and are considered a marker of unresectability. Cytology positive for malignancy on a thoracentesis is indicative of an unresectable malignancy of the lung.

6-C. Oat cell carcinoma of the lung is the classic form of small cell carcinoma (SCCA). SCCAs of the lung are generally considered unresectable, and are treated primarily with chemotherapy. Positive mediastinal nodes are also an indicator of unresectability. A small number of small SCCA located in the lung periphery with little or no nodal involvement may additionally be treated with resection of the primary lesion. Radiation therapy alone would be inadequate therapy.

7-D. Symptomatic hamartomas can be treated with simple wedge resection of the lesion. Some asymptomatic hamartomas found incidentally on radiograph may be treated with observation and serial films to evaluate for changes in the lesion suggestive of malignancy but symptomatic lesions should be resected. Bronchoscopic resection would be inadequate treatment.

8-E. Treatment of a pulmonary abscess is frequently nonsurgical with administration of intravenous antibiotics and chest physiotherapy to facilitate drainage of the abscess. However, patients with recurrent pneumonia should be suspected of having an obstructive lesion causing a postobstructive pneumonia or abscess as in this setting. Bronchoscopy would allow for evaluation of a potential obstructive lesion. Surgical resection, surgical drainage, or lobectomy are generally not required for abscesses.

9-B. Diagnosis of mediastinal masses before planning resection is important particularly in the setting of lymphoma, which is frequently treated without surgical resection. Lymphomas in the mediastinum most frequently occur in the anterior mediastinum and are mostly T cell lymphomas. Treatment of mediastinal lymphomas with concurrent disease in other sites is with systemic chemotherapy with or without radiation therapy. Mediastinal disease that causes significant symptoms (e.g., shortness of breath from airway obstruction) may rarely require surgical intervention.

10-D. Myasthenia gravis may represent a paraneoplastic syndrome of thymomas. It is estimated that 10%–75% of patients with a thymoma will develop myasthenia gravis, while only 10% of patients with myasthenia gravis will have a thymoma. Other rare paraneoplastic syndromes associated with thymoma include red cell aplasia and hypogammaglobulinemia. If a thymoma is present, thymectomy may relieve symptoms in many patients. Myasthenia gravis is associated with the presence of antibody to acetylcholine receptor rather than acetylcholine. Thymomas may also be malignant in more than 25% of patients, thus resection is always indicated.

11-A. Rarely, the thyroid gland may migrate into the superior or anterior mediastinum during embryologic migration. In addition, thyroid goiter may be large enough to extend into the mediastinum. This may present as a large mediastinal mass during evaluation. The diffuse lymphocytic infiltrate with normal germinal centers is a characteristic finding of Hashimoto's thyroiditis, which is the most common cause of noniatrogenic hypothyroidism and goiter. This finding does not represent a lymphoma.

12-E. Initial episodes of a spontaneous pneumothorax in an otherwise healthy patient may be treated with simple chest tube thoracostomy alone; however, there are some indications for further therapy given the high risk of recurrence after an initial episode (~50%). Such indications include patients in which a pneumothorax could result in potential disaster, including individuals that work at altitudes, such as airline pilots, mountain climbers, etc. Appropriate treatment in this setting would include chest tube placement with definitive treatment of the bullous disease with wedge resection and subsequent mechanical pleurodesis. Mechanical pleurodesis involves delicate scraping of the visceral and parietal pleura to produce an inflammatory reaction that eventually allows for permanent apposition of the pleura. Pleurodesis alone is inadequate therapy without resection of the bullous disease.

13-D. Although an overall elevation in the white blood cell (WBC) count of pleural fluid may indicate a chylothorax, a high WBC count (over 15,000 cells/μL) consisting predominantly of polymorphonuclear leukocytes is consistent with the presence of an empyema. Positive Sudan red staining and the presence of chylomicra is consistent with a diagnosis of chylothorax rather than empyema. The specific gravity of the fluid is also a nonspecific marker, although the specific gravity of fluid from an empyema is typically higher than 1.018.

14-C. Although direct biopsy of the lesion is important, the presence of an associated pleural effusion should raise the suspicion of a malignant pleural effusion. Thoracentesis and cytologic analysis of this fluid may be diagnostic without having to perform a biopsy or resection of the lung lesion. The presence of a malignant pleural effusion also indicates a T4 lesion, which is considered an unresectable lesion. Mediastinoscopy and biopsy of enlarged paratracheal nodes would not be the initial step and would generally not be necessary if a malignant pleural effusion is identified.

15-D. The choice between a mechanical valve and a tissue valve is based on the relative advantages and disadvantages of each type of valve. Patients with a longer life expectancy often receive mechanical valves because they generally are more durable than tissue valves. Mechanical valves, on the other hand, require life-long anticoagulation therapy with coumarin (Coumadin) with the associated risks of bleeding diathesis (e.g., intraventricular hemorrhage) while tissue valves do not require long-term anticoagulation. Neither valve requires administration of immunosuppressive therapy following insertion.

3

Pediatric

R. Cartland Burns

I. Anomalies of the Chest and Mediastinum

A. Chest wall deformities

1. **Pectus excavatum** (funnel chest)

   —is characterized **by posterior displacement** of the inferior **sternum** and xiphoid related to abnormal development of the costal cartilage.

   a. This **defect is often corrected** to relieve psychologic distress associated with the cosmetic appearance of the defect.

   b. The **defect is occasionally associated** with cardiovascular and respiratory compromise and decreased exercise tolerance.

   c. **Surgical correction**

      —involves **sternal osteotomy.**

      —sometimes requires placement of a temporary metal strut to stabilize the deformed sternum in its new anterior position.

2. **Pectus carinatum** (pigeon chest)

   —is **characterized** by **anterior displacement of the sternum.**

   —Like excavatum, early surgical repair (after 6 years of age) is generally performed to prevent psychological distress in affected individuals.

B. Pulmonary sequestration

—is an anomaly in which there is a portion of lung tissue that has **no communication with the tracheobronchial tree.**

1. The **blood supply** usually arises from anomalous vessels, frequently from below the **diaphragm.**

2. **Intralobar sequestrations** are contained wholly within normal surrounding lung tissue.

   —These are rarely associated with other anomalies.

3. **Extralobar sequestration** is completely separate from normal lung parenchyma, and may be below the diaphragm.

—These are more commonly associated with other anomalies (e.g., diaphragmatic hernia).

4. **Manifestations of sequestration** may include

—abnormal chest radiograph.

—**recurrent pneumonia.**

—**respiratory compromise.**

5. **Treatment**

—requires excision, with care taken to identify and ligate the anomalous blood supply.

C. **Congenital cystic adenomatoid malformation (CCAM)**

—is characterized by the development of bronchial structures at the expense of alveolar structures.

1. **These lesions**

—may be microcystic or macrocystic.

—**may compromise development of normal lung tissue.**

2. **Prenatal ultrasound**

—may be diagnostic, although infants may present with respiratory compromise or recurrent infection.

3. **Fetal hydrops**

—may develop, and is associated with a 90% mortality rate.

4. **Treatment**

—is **surgical excision of the involved lobe.**

D. **Congenital lobar emphysema**

—is an **overexpansion of the airways** of a segment of lung.

1. **Emphysema occurs** because of abnormal bronchial cartilage, resulting in air trapping.

—Overexpansion may progress and impinge on normal lung tissue.

2. The **left upper and right middle lobes** are most commonly affected.

3. This may **present** with respiratory distress in the first few days of life or may be asymptomatic until many months later.

4. The **male to female ratio is 3:1.**

5. **Diagnosis**

—is usually made by plain chest radiograph.

6. **Treatment**

—is by **resection of the affected lobe.**

E. **Bronchogenic cysts**

—usually present as a **mediastinal cystic mass** filled with milky mucoid liquid.

1. These **cysts**

    —are lined by cuboidal or columnar epithelium and mucous glands.

    —may produce **symptoms** because of **compression of normal structures.**

    —may **become infected** if there is bronchial communication.

2. A **chest radiograph**

    —is often suggestive, with chest computed tomography (CT) confirming the diagnosis.

3. **Treatment**

    —involves cyst resection.

    —Intrapulmonary cysts may require lobectomy.

F. **Tracheoesophageal fistula and esophageal atresia**

1. The **pathogenesis of these anomalies** is uncertain, although they probably occur at the fourth to fifth week of embryonic development.

2. The 5 **types** of **tracheoesophageal anomalies**

    are outlined in **Figure 3.1.**

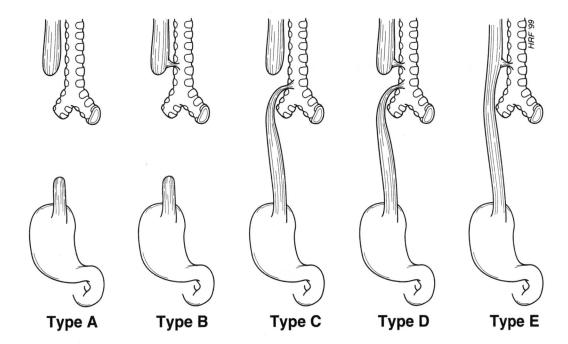

Type A   **Type B**   **Type C**   **Type D**   **Type E**

Figure 3.1. The five types of tracheoesophageal fistulae or esophageal atresias:
Type A: 6%, atresia alone, no fistula; small stomach, gasless abdomen
Type B: 2%, proximal tracheoesophageal fistula; no distal fistula; small stomach, gasless abdomen
Type C: 85%, most common abnormality
Type D: 1%, proximal and distal fistulas
Type E: ("H"-type tracheoesophageal fistula) 6%, no esophageal atresia
(Adapted with permission from Beasly SW: Esophageal Atresia and Tracheoesophageal Fistula. In *Surgery of Infants and Children: Scientific Principles and Practice.* Edited by Oldham KT, Colombani PM, Foglia RP. Philadelphia, Lippincott, 1997, p 1024.)

3. **Tracheoesophageal fistulae** are frequently associated with other anomalies including the **VACTERL constellation** of anomalies:

—*v*ertebral anomalies (hemivertebrae).

—*a*norectal anomalies (imperforate anus).

—*c*ardiac defects.

—*t*racheoesophageal anomalies.

—*r*enal (genitourinary) deformities.

—*l*imb deformities (radial anomalies).

4. **Survival is related to**

—**birth weight.**

—the presence of **cardiac anomalies.**

5. **Presentation and diagnosis**
   a. **Newborns** may present with
      —excessive drooling.
      —choking.
      —coughing.
      —regurgitation with first feeding.
   b. **Inability to pass an orogastric tube into the stomach**
      —is **diagnostic** of **esophageal atresia.**
   c. **Absence of stomach air**
      —suggests pure **esophageal atresia** without distal fistula.

6. **Preoperative assessment**

   —**for other associated anomalies (e.g., cardiac, renal)** is essential.

7. **Treatment and follow-up**
   a. The **tracheoesophageal fistula** is **repaired** and esophago-esophagostomy performed if the length is adequate, via a right extrapleural thoracotomy.
   b. **Postoperative esophageal leak** may occur and can be treated with chest drainage.
   c. **Close follow-up is needed** because many of these children have **gastroesophageal reflux and may develop anastomotic strictures** that require dilation.

G. **Mediastinal masses** (see Chapter 2, Table 2-2)

II. Gastrointestinal Disorders

A. **Hypertrophic pyloric stenosis**
   1. **Pyloric stenosis**

      —**results** from hypertrophy of the pyloric muscle.
   2. The **incidence**

      —is greatest in **first-born males** (male:female ratio of 5:1).

3. **Children**

    —**present** with **progressive, nonbilious vomiting (which may be projectile) between 2–8 weeks.**

4. The **diagnosis** is made by

    —**palpation of pyloric "tumor"** or "olive."

    —**ultrasound** measurement of enlarged pylorus ($\geq$ 4 mm thick, $\geq$ 14 mm long).

5. **Affected infants frequently present** with

    —**hypokalemic, hypochloremic metabolic alkalosis.**

    —paradoxical aciduria.

6. **Electrolyte disturbances** should be corrected before operation.

    —These infants are given 10% dextrose solution because they are prone to hypoglycemia as a result of their small glycogen stores.

7. **Treatment** of choice

    —is **surgical correction** via a **pyloromyotomy** (Ramstedt).

B. **Intestinal malrotation (Figure 3.2)**

    —results from **failure of the normal 270° counterclockwise rotation** of the duodenojejunal and cecocolic loops during fetal development (week 10–12).

1. The narrow mesenteric stalk predisposes the midgut to volvulus with obstruction of the upper gastrointestinal tract and vascular compromise of the superior mesenteric artery.

2. **Children with malrotation usually present** in the **first month of life with bilious emesis** caused by duodenal obstruction.

    a. It should be noted that bilious emesis in a child younger than 2 months old should be considered a **surgical emergency** until proven otherwise.

    b. Infants may present with **acute midgut volvulus and ischemic bowel.**

3. The **diagnosis**

    —is based on clinical suspicion.

    —should be confirmed by contrast upper gastrointestinal series.

4. **Early surgical correction**

    —is **essential** because of the risk of volvulus and ischemia.

5. The classic **Ladd's procedure** includes four stages:

    a. **Counterclockwise detorsion**

        —of the midgut

    b. **Division of bands**

        —between the cecum and posterior abdominal wall in the right upper quadrant (**Ladd's bands**)

    c. **Release of adhesions**

        —between the cecum and duodenum to widen the mesentery.

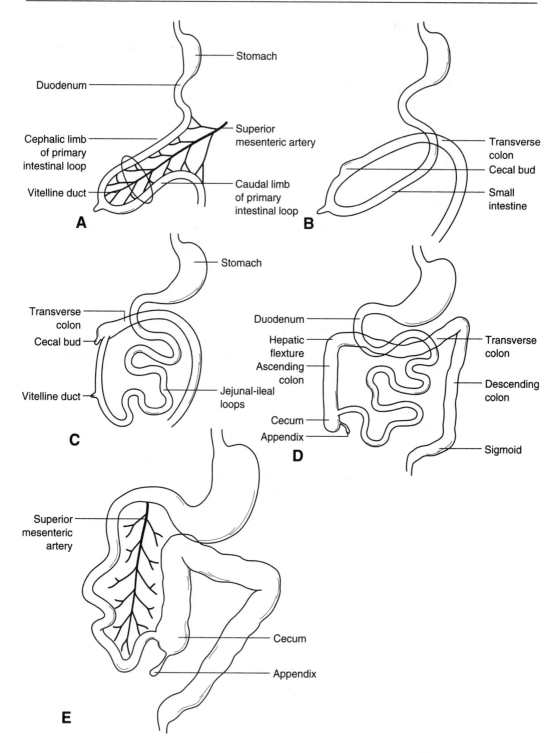

Figure 3.2. Normal bowel rotation and nonrotation. (*A*) Lateral view of the primitive intestinal loop before rotation. (*B*) Lateral view of the primitive intestinal loop after 180° counterclockwise rotation. (*C*) Anterior view of the intestinal loops after 270° counterclockwise rotation. (*D*) Intestinal loops in normal final position. (*E*) Nonrotation of the intestinal loop with the cecum and appendix to the left of the superior mesenteric artery. (Adapted with permission from Sadler TW: Digestive System. In *Langman's Medical Embryology,* 5th ed. Edited by Sadler TW. Baltimore, Williams & Wilkins, 1985, pp 236–237.)

    d. Placement of the cecum

        —in the left upper quadrant while directing the duodenum down the right side of the abdomen, with performance of an appendectomy.

C. Duodenal atresia

    —occurs as a result of failure of recanalization of the duodenum during weeks 8–10 of fetal development.

    1. Other anomalies frequently occur, particularly **trisomy 21 (Down syndrome).**

        —Cardiac, renal, and other gastrointestinal anomalies (e.g., annular pancreas) may be present.

    2. Atresia occurs in 3 types, as depicted in **Figure 3.3.**

    3. Presentation

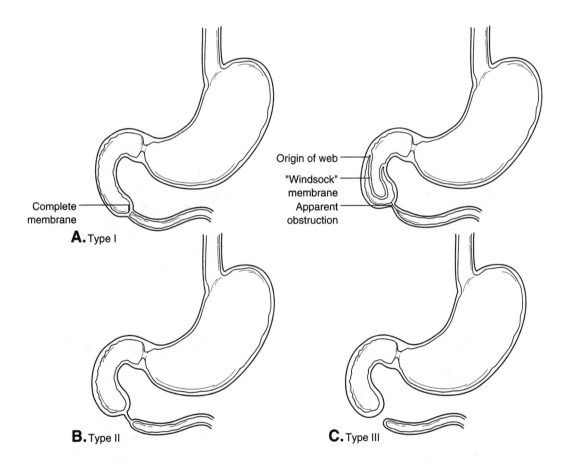

Figure 3.3. The three types of duodenal atresias. (*A*) All variations of Type I lesions contain a luminal membrane. Type I lesions may present as a windsock deformity with a duodenal web protruding downstream into the lumen, making the membrane difficult to identify. (*B*) Type II lesions contain a small fibrotic band between the proximal and distal segments. (*C*) Type III lesions are complete without any connection between the two segments. (Adapted with permission from Magnuson DK, Schwartz MZ: Stomach and Duodenum. In *Surgery of Infants and Children: Scientific Principles and Practice.* Edited by Oldham KT, Colombani PM, Foglia RP. Philadelphia, Lippincott, 1997, pp 1149–1150.)

a. **Polyhydramnios**

—may be seen in utero with resultant premature labor.

b. **Newborns begin to vomit shortly after birth.**

—The **emesis is usually bilious** because the obstruction is distal to the bile duct in 80% of cases.

c. The **abdomen** is **not distended**

—because the distal bowel is not distended.

d. **Abdominal films**

—show a characteristic **double bubble sign** of duodenal obstruction **(Figure 3.4).**

(1) Distal air is usually absent.

(2) Upper gastrointestinal series may help to differentiate atresia from malrotation if the clinical findings are not clear.

4. **Treatment**

—initially involves adequate resuscitation and evaluation for other associated congenital anomalies.

5. **Surgery**

a. **Duodenal webs (Type I)**

—**are fenestrated,** with care to avoid the ampulla of Vater.

b. An **atresia with discontinuity**

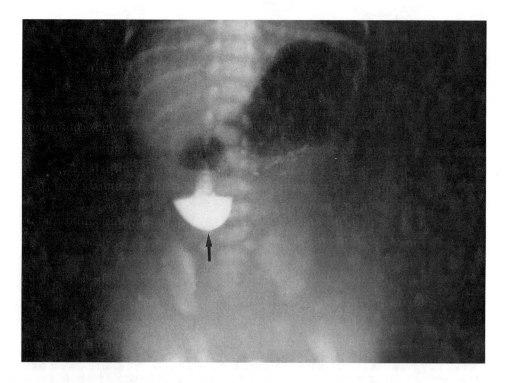

Figure 3.4. Double bubble sign associated with duodenal atresia. Note air trapped in both the stomach and duodenal bulb. The white density is barium in the descending duodenum with abrupt termination at the level of the atresia (*arrow*). (Reprinted with permission from Daffner RH: Abdominal Radiographs. In *Clinical Radiology, The Essentials,* 2nd ed. Edited by Daffner RH. Baltimore, Lippincott Williams & Wilkins, 1999, p 263.)

—of the duodenum should be directly anastomosed (**duodenoduodenostomy**) if possible.

c. **Return of gastrointestinal function**

—may be slow to develop and children should be supported with parenteral nutrition during this time.

D. Small bowel atresia

1. **Congenital occlusion of the small bowel lumen**

—results in intestinal obstruction.

2. **Small bowel atresia**

—is caused by a **late intrauterine mesenteric vascular insult.**

3. **There are four types** of small bowel atresia

—ranging from simple mucosal atresia with intact muscularis and mesentery (Type I) to multiple atresias with the appearance of a string of sausages (Type IV) with associated mesenteric defects.

4. **Patients may present** with

—maternal hydramnios.

—bilious emesis.

—variable abdominal distension correlating with the level of the atresia.

—Most of these children **do not pass meconium,** although they may pass small amounts of stool initially.

5. **Plain abdominal radiographs**

—**reveal dilated loops of small intestine** with air fluid levels proximal to the atresia, with no gas noted distal to the atresia.

6. **Preoperative treatment**

—involves **fluid resuscitation and gastrointestinal decompression.**

7. **Resection of the atretic segment or segments**

—is performed with subsequent end-to-end anastomosis of the remaining bowel if possible.

8. **Survival**

—approaches 100% in children without other serious anomalies.

E. Imperforate anus

—occurs in 1/5,000 live births.

—is **more common in males.**

1. The **diagnosis**

—is made by **thorough physical examination** of the newborn.

2. **Lesions are classified** as either **high or low.**

—This depends on the location of the distal portion of **rectal remnant in relation to the levator muscle (Figure 3.5).**

—Associated anomalies should be evaluated (e.g., renal anomalies, tethered cord).

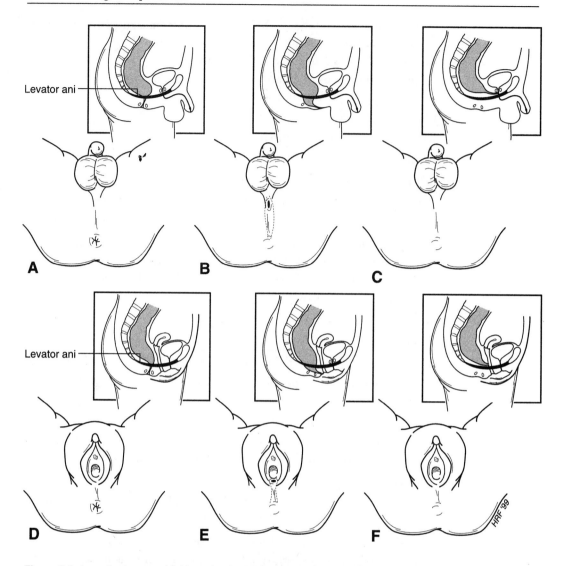

Figure 3.5. Imperforate anus. (*A*) Normal male. (*B*) Male with low imperforate lesion and anterior subcutaneous fistula. (*C*) Male with high lesion. Rectum ends in posterior urethra. (*D*) Normal female. (*E*) Female with low imperforate anus and fistula at vaginal opening. (*F*) Female with high lesion. Rectum ends in upper vagina. (Adapted with permission from Coran AG, Behrendt DM, Weintraub WH, Lee DC: *Surgery of the Neonate.* Boston, Little, Brown, 1978, p 181.)

3. **Treatment**

   —depends on the level of the lesion.

   a. **High lesions**

      —**require colostomy** in the newborn period with delayed posterior sagittal anorectoplasty (Peña procedure).

   b. **Low lesions**

      —with perineal fistulae may be treated with limited posterior anoplasty in the newborn period.

4. **Postoperative anal dilations**

   —are performed to avoid anal stricture.

5. **Careful attention must be paid** to the management of constipation in these children because most are prone to constipation.

F. Hirschsprung disease

—is caused by **failure of craniocaudal progression of neural crest cells** into the myenteric (Auerbach) and submucosal (Meissner) plexus.

1. **Presentation**
   a. **Patients most commonly present** with
      —**failure to pass meconium** within the first 24–48 hours of life.
   b. **Others may present** with
      —**chronic constipation** usually by age 2–3 years.
   c. Three to five percent of patients may have associated Down syndrome or trisomy 21.

2. **Physical examination** may reveal
   —**abdominal distension.**
   —explosive release of watery stool on rectal examination.

3. **Radiologic studies**
   —include barium enema.
   —may show a spastic distal rectum or sigmoid colon with proximal dilated colon and a **tapered zone between the two regions, called the transition zone.**

4. **Rectal biopsy**
   —is the key to **diagnosis.**
   —Pathologic findings include the **absence of normal ganglion cells** and hypertrophic preganglionic nerve trunks.

5. **Intraoperative serial biopsies**
   —are performed to define the level of affected bowel.

6. **Once the level of diseased bowel is noted**
   —the **proximal end is brought to the skin as a stoma,** and the distal end is closed and left in place for later resection.

7. **Definitive surgical management** is designed to
   —**remove the diseased segment** of bowel.
   —create an **anastomosis between the normal bowel and the anus.**
   a. Three such operations include Swenson, Soave, and Duhamel procedures.
   b. This procedure may now be performed in the newborn period.

8. **Hirschsprung enterocolitis**
   —may be rapidly progressive.
   —is **manifested** by explosive, **foul-smelling watery diarrhea** in a child with abdominal distension and either suspected or diagnosed Hirschsprung disease.
   a. **Children with this type of enterocolitis**
      —may be lethargic.

—may have **systemic signs of sepsis.**

b. **Treatment** includes

—broad spectrum antibiotics.

—rectal irrigation whenever suspected, because the disease carries a **mortality rate of as high as 30%.**

G. **Intussusception**

—is the **invagination of one portion of the intestine into the lumen of the distal adjoining segment.**

1. **Patients usually present** between 3 months and 3 years of age with **paroxysms of violent abdominal pain.**

   a. **The child may appear lethargic** or apathetic following these episodes.

   b. **Once the intussusception has persisted** for several hours, the child will begin to

      —pass **bloody stools or "currant jelly" stools.**

      —**vomit.**

      —develop volume depletion.

2. **Pathologic lead points may be identified,** such as

   —**enlarged Peyer's patches.**

   —Meckel diverticulum.

   —Henoch-Schönlein purpura (submucosal hematoma).

   —lymphoma.

3. **Physical examination may reveal**

   —a lethargic child with right-sided abdominal tenderness.

   —possibly a mass in the right upper quadrant (Dance's sign).

4. **Initial treatment**

   —should involve **fluid resuscitation.**

5. **Hydrostatic or pneumatic reduction with barium or air**

   —can successfully confirm the **diagnosis.**

   —can **successfully treat the intussusception nonoperatively 90% of the time.**

6. **Surgery is indicated** in the setting of

   —peritonitis.

   —perforation.

   —failed reduction.

7. **Surgical reduction** involves squeezing the intussuscepted portion, pushing from the distal end.

   —The bowel should never be pulled from the proximal end.

   a. A **thorough search** should be conducted for a pathologic lead point.

   b. If compromised **bowel is identified, it should be resected and primary anastomosis performed.**

8. **Recurrence rates** of

—10%–20% occur following nonoperative reduction.

—approximately 3% after surgical reduction are reported.

H. Meckel diverticulum

—(see *BRS General Surgery,* Chapter 13 VII B)

I. Necrotizing enterocolitis (NEC)

—presents in newborns (younger than 2 weeks old).

—affects preterm infants more frequently than term infants.

—is **characterized** by **mucosal ischemia that can progress to full-thickness necrosis.**

—is associated with an overall mortality rate of approximately 20%.

1. The **etiology**

—of this disease is currently unknown.

2. **Risk factors** for development of NEC include

—prematurity.

—hypoxia or hypotension.

—anemia or polycythemia.

—sepsis.

—hyperosmolar feedings.

—intracranial hemorrhage.

—maternal cocaine use.

3. The **diagnosis should be considered**

—in any at-risk newborn with suggestive signs or symptoms of disease.

4. **Findings** may include

—**lethargy.**

—**respiratory decompensation.**

—**abdominal distension.**

—**vomiting.**

—**diarrhea.**

—**blood per rectum.**

—**high gastric residuals** after enteral feedings.

5. **Plain radiographs of the abdomen** may be diagnostic, demonstrating

—pneumatosis intestinalis.

—free air.

—portal vein air.

6. **Initial treatment** involves

—**bowel rest** (nothing by mouth [NPO], orogastric suction, **parenteral nutrition support**).

—adequate **fluid resuscitation.**

—**intravenous (IV) antibiotics.**

7. The **presence of peritonitis** or signs of perforation require laparotomy and surgical resection of necrotic bowel or drainage of the peritoneal cavity.

J. **Meconium ileus**

—occurs from the inspissation of **abnormally thick and viscous meconium** in children with **cystic fibrosis.**

1. **Meconium ileus**

—**occurs** in approximately 10% of children with **cystic fibrosis.**

2. **Usual presentation**

—is that of **small bowel obstruction** (abdominal distension, bilious emesis) within the **first 1–2 days of life.**

3. **Plain radiographs**

—reveal dilated loops of bowel without air fluid levels because the meconium is too thick to separate from the bowel wall.

—A **characteristic ground glass or soap bubble appearance** is noted.

4. The **diagnosis is confirmed** by

—**water-soluble contrast enema** that demonstrates microcolon (caused by lack of use).

—inspissated pellets of meconium in the terminal ileum.

5. **Therapy** may be **nonsurgical**

—**with either water-soluble contrast enema, or N-acetylcysteine enema to loosen the inspissated meconium.**

6. **If nonoperative measures fail,** then laparotomy is indicated.

7. **Operative measures** include

—injection of N-acetylcysteine into the affected bowel, manipulating the pellets into the distal bowel.

—enterotomy to remove the meconium, if necessary.

8. **Complications of meconium ileus** include

—**intestinal perforation that may occur prenatally,** resulting in meconium pseudocyst or peritonitis and requiring laparotomy.

III. Congenital Defects of the Biliary Tree

A. **Biliary atresia**

—is a **congenital obliteration of the extrahepatic or intrahepatic biliary tree** with an unknown etiology.

1. This atresia is the **most common cause** of **neonatal jaundice** that requires surgery.

—**Persistent jaundice in newborns** lasting over 2 weeks is suggestive of atresia.

2. The **atretic biliary tree** is often demonstrated with

—ultrasound.

—cholangiography.

—nuclear scanning.

3. A **liver biopsy** may **reveal**

—periportal fibrosis.

—bile plugging.

—eventual cirrhosis.

4. **Treatment** of isolated extrahepatic biliary atresia

—is via a modified Roux-en-Y hepatoportoenterostomy (Kasai procedure).

5. **Most patients eventually require hepatic transplantation** for definitive therapy.

B. **Choledochal cysts**

—(see *BRS General Surgery,* Chapter 16 IX A 2)

C. **Pancreatic divisum and annular pancreas**

—(see *BRS General Surgery,* Chapter 17 II D)

IV. Abdominal Wall Defects

A. **Umbilical hernia**

1. **Umbilical hernias**

—**result from** a congenital fascial wall defect around the umbilicus that is **covered by normal skin.**

—**occur** much more frequently in **African-American infants.**

2. **Prematurity is a significant risk factor** for the occurrence of these hernias.

3. **Most will close spontaneously** in the first 3 years of life.

4. **Indications for surgery** include

—**incarceration.**

—**pain.**

—**failure to close by 3–4 years of age.**

B. **Omphalocele** (Table 3-1)

—is an umbilical defect that occurs because **the lateral folds of the body wall fail to close.**

1. **This defect**

—may contain abdominal contents, including liver in nearly 50% of cases.

Table 3-1. Omphalocele Versus Gastroschisis

	Omphalocele	Gastroschisis
Description	Incomplete fusion of lateral folds of body wall	Rupture of cord membrane at skin attachment
Sac	Covered by avascular sac of peritoneum and amniotic membrane (Wharton's jelly)	No hernia sac; bowel are exposed to amniotic fluid, appearing as inflamed mass
Diagnosis	Obvious at physical examination if not diagnosed prenatally	Prenatal ultrasound; physical examination reveals herniated viscera at the right side of the umbilicus
Associated anomalies		
Gastrointestinal	Few gastrointestinal anomalies	Gastrointestinal anomalies common (15%)
Other	Frequently associated with cardiac and CNS anomalies (35%–80%), many of which are lethal	Rarely associated with non-gastrointestinal anomalies
Liver involvement	Attached to defect	Uninvolved
Rotation	May be associated with normal rotation or non-rotation of the intestines	Almost always associated with nonrotation of the intestines
Survival	60% overall, related to presence of other anomalies (e.g., cardiac, CNS defects)	Well over 80%

CNS = central nervous system.

> —has a **high rate of associated anomalies (e.g., cardiac and CNS defects).**
> 2. **Diagnosis**
>   a. The **abdominal wall defect**
>   —is seen protruding into the umbilical cord with the vessels arising from the top of the lesion.
>   b. The **sac**
>   —**may be intact,** with normal-appearing intestines within.
>   —**may be ruptured,** with the viscera exposed.
>   c. **These defects may be** small (4 cm) or large (up to 12 cm).
> 3. **Treatment**
>   a. The **intact sac** should be covered with sterile saline-soaked gauze.
>   —The child must be kept warm while other anomalies are sought.
>   —The small intact omphalocele can be repaired primarily when the patient is stable.
>   —Larger intact lesions can be covered with an antibiotic solution and allowed to epithelialize.

   b. If the **sac is ruptured**
      —the viscera are covered with sterile saline-soaked gauze while the child is prepared for **emergent repair.**

C. **Gastroschisis** (see Table 3-1)
   —is the **herniation of abdominal contents** to the right of the umbilical cord.
   1. **Presentation**
      a. **Because the viscera are exposed** to the amniotic fluid, the result is a **matted mass of inflamed bowel.**
      b. **Stomach and small bowel** are frequently herniated, and the liver is rarely involved.
   2. **The child rarely has other anomalies**
      —although small bowel atresia may occur due to vascular compromise at the umbilical ring.
   3. **Diagnosis** (see Table 3-1)
      —The **bowel is covered in a gelatinous, inflammatory mass.**
   4. **Initial treatment** requires
      —covering the bowel with saline-soaked gauze.
      —elevating the intestine to avoid venous congestion.
   5. **Great care must be given** to keeping the child warm in preparation for emergent laparotomy for closure.
   6. **To permit primary closure,** the **abdominal wall musculature** is usually adequate.
      a. **If closure requires undue pressure** (compromising ventilation), then the hernia defect is widened and a silo device is sutured to the margins.
      b. Once the **abdominal contents are easily reduced,** the silo is removed and the fascia is closed.
   7. **Survival** is well over 80%.
      —Delayed motility, however, may require long-term parenteral nutrition.

D. **Inguinal hernia**
   —in a child is an indirect inguinal hernia resulting from a **patent processus vaginalis,** which normally obliterates during fetal development.
   1. **Incidence**
      —is 3%–5% in term infants.
      —is as high as **15% in premature infants.**
      —**Boys are affected six times as often as girls are.**
   2. **Affected sides**
      —Right side is affected in 60% of cases.
      —Left side (30%).
      —Both sides (10%).

—The right processus vaginalis obliterates later than the left.

3. On **physical examination**

—a firm smooth mass extending up to the level of the internal inguinal ring is noted.

   a. The **mass may be tender** and may vary with crying.

   b. **Extension to the internal ring differentiates a hernia from a hydrocele.**

   (1) A **hydrocele** represents a collection of fluid within the tunica vaginalis that may or may not communicate with peritoneum depending on the patency of the processus vaginalis.

   (2) In children, both **hernias and fluid-filled hydroceles** will usually **transilluminate.**

4. **Initial treatment**

—should include manual reduction if possible, in the absence of peritoneal signs.

5. **Definitive treatment**

—is by **operative closure of the processus vaginalis** at the earliest convenient time.

   a. **In infants under 1 year of age and most females**

   —both groins are frequently explored because of the risk of **bilateral occurrence.**

   b. **During open repair of a unilateral symptomatic hernia**

   —the asymptomatic side may be explored laparoscopically from the symptomatic side.

   c. **In boys over 1 year of age**

   —the symptomatic side only is repaired, because there is a small risk that a patent processus vaginalis is present and has not yet become clinically apparent.

E. **Congenital diaphragmatic hernia (CDH)**

—occurs in 1/2000–5000 live births and is more common in males.

—**Eighty percent occur on the left side.**

1. The **Bochdalek hernia**

—is most common.

—occurs in the **posterolateral position** where the septum transversum fails to fuse with the pleuroperitoneal folds during the eighth week of development.

2. The **Morgagni hernia** is a rare defect that occurs in a retrosternal position. **Associated anomalies occur** in approximately 50% of these children.

—They are most commonly **cardiac or neural tube defects.**

3. **Diagnosis**

—is frequently (80%–90%) made by **prenatal ultrasound.**

4. **These patients present** with **respiratory distress,** usually shortly after birth.

—The respiratory distress is related to abnormal development of the ipsilateral lung.

    a. The **resultant pulmonary hypoplasia**

      —may lead to **pulmonary hypertension.**

    b. A **scaphoid abdomen**

      —is also a characteristic finding.

5. Chest radiograph

—shows the intestine to be located in the chest.

—may demonstrate mediastinal shift.

6. The patient should be stabilized and undergo echocardiogram and renal ultrasound prior to operative repair.

    a. Infants suffering from **respiratory failure**

      —**may be candidates for extracorporeal membrane oxygenation (ECMO).**

    b. **Operative repair**

      —is undertaken once the child is stable, because operative repair is of secondary importance to the respiratory support.

      —includes the reduction of the hernia contents and repair of the diaphragm defect either primarily or with a prosthetic patch.

    c. **The survival rate**

      —is approximately 60%.

F. Prune belly syndrome (Eagle-Barrett syndrome)

—is a rare congenital absence or **hypoplasia of the abdominal musculature.**

—The **complete triad of symptoms** also includes **urinary tract abnormalities** with a dilated urinary system and **bilateral cryptorchidism.**

V. Neoplasms

A. Neuroblastoma

—is a tumor of **neural crest origin** that may arise in any location along the **sympathetic chain** from the neck to the pelvis (e.g., posterior mediastinum, adrenals, pelvis, neck).

1. The **most common site of origin** is the **adrenal medulla.**

2. Epidemiology

    a. Neuroblastoma is the **most common solid abdominal malignancy** of the newborn, with an incidence of 1/8,000.

    b. **Ninety percent present** before 8 years of age, with **most presenting in children younger than 2 years.**

3. Presentation

    a. **Patients present** with

      —**abdominal mass (50%–75%).**

      —**hypertension (25%).**

    b. This **tumor may be associated** with

—an autoimmune-mediated **opsoclonus-myoclonus (dancing eyes) and unsteady gait,** usually in younger patients.

c. **Orbital metastases present** with

—bilateral ecchymoses or proptosis without a history of trauma.

4. **Diagnosis**

a. **CT scan** helps to identify

—the origin of the mass.

—the relationship to other organs.

—characteristic encasement rather than invasion of vascular structures.

b. **Plain radiographs**

—may show **stippled calcifications** within the tumor.

c. Of **these tumors,** 90% secrete high levels of **catecholamine** or derivatives.

d. Twenty-four hour **urine collection** may reveal

—elevated **homovanillic acid** (HVA; product of dopamine).

—elevated **vanillylmandelic acid** (VMA; product of epinephrine and norepinephrine).

5. The **International Neuroblastoma Staging System**

—is outlined in **Table 3-2.**

6. **Prognosis**

—N-*myc* proto-oncogene amplification (over 10 copies) connotes a **poor prognosis.**

7. **Treatment**

a. **Surgical excision** of the tumor

—is the primary therapy for resectable lesions.

b. **Initially unresectable tumors**

—may become resectable following chemotherapy.

Table 3-2. International Neuroblastoma Staging System

Stage	Characteristics
1	Tumor confined to area of origin with complete excision
2A	Unilateral tumor with incomplete excision and negative nodes
2B	Unilateral tumor with complete or incomplete excision and positive regional nodes and negative contralateral nodes
3	Tumor crosses midline or unilateral tumor with positive contralateral nodes or midline tumor with bilateral nodal involvement
4	Disseminated tumor to bone, bone marrow, liver, distant nodes, or other organs (except as noted in 4S)
4S	Localized primary tumor as defined by stage 1 or 2 with dissemination limited to liver, skin, and bone marrow.

B. **Wilms tumor (nephroblastoma)**
   1. **Wilms tumors** are **composed of three cell types:**
      —blastema.

      —stroma.

      —epithelium.
   2. These tumors may **be associated** with

      —**Beckwith-Wiedemann syndrome.**

      —hemihypertrophy.

      —cryptorchidism.

      —Drash syndrome.

      —aniridia.
   3. The **mean age at diagnosis is 3 years.**

      —Approximately **10% of tumors are bilateral.**
   4. The **typical presentation**

      —is that of an otherwise healthy child found to have a **large, nontender, fixed abdominal mass** that rarely crosses the midline.

      —Patients may have **hematuria or hypertension.**
   5. **Diagnosis**
      a. A **chest radiograph**

         —is frequently used to screen for lung metastasis.
      b. **Abdominal CT**

         —typically demonstrates the site of the lesion usually with replacement of renal parenchyma (not displacement as seen in neuroblastoma).

         —also **characterizes any involvement of the inferior vena cava via the renal vein,** and the presence of metastases in the contralateral kidney.
   6. The **National Wilms Tumor Study group staging system**

      —is outlined in **Table 3-3.**
   7. **Treatment**
      a. **Surgical management**

         —**allows for complete resection** of the tumor and **accurate staging** for adjuvant therapy planning.
      b. **Peritoneal implants**

         —are sought and biopsied if found.
      c. The **contralateral kidney is fully evaluated**

         —by visual inspection and palpation.
      d. **Ipsilateral nephroureterectomy**

         —is performed with great care to avoid tumor rupture, because this increases the stage of the tumor.
      e. If **venous extension** is found

         —the **tumor thrombus is carefully extracted from the vein.**

Table 3-3. National Wilms Tumor Study Group Staging System

Stage	Description	2-Year Survival for Favorable Tumors
I	Tumor confined to ipsilateral kidney and completely excised without tumor rupture	95%
II	Tumor extends beyond kidney but is completely excised; perirenal or venous extension may be present; localized tumor spill may have occurred	91%
III	Residual tumor remains after resection; may include nodal metastases, diffuse tumor spill, or peritoneal implants; also includes tumor biopsy without resection	90%
IV	Hematogenous distant metastases	43%
V	Bilateral disease	76%

    f. **All enlarged lymph nodes**
        —are sampled as well.

   8. **Adjuvant therapy**
       —is an important part of the treatment of Wilms tumor.
       a. **All children with Wilms tumor except stage I tumors weighing less than 500 g**
           —**receive actinomycin and vincristine.**
       b. **Patients with stage II and higher**
           —receive doxorubicin in addition.
       c. **Children** with **stage III and higher**
           —**also receive abdominal radiation.**

   9. The **prognosis** is related to the stage of disease and the histologic findings.
       —Unfavorable histologic features include anaplasia with multipolar mitotic figures and nuclear enlargement with hyperchromasia.

 C. **Hepatoblastoma**
     —is the most common malignant liver tumor in children.

   1. The **majority of tumors** are **found before age 18 months.**
   2. There is **an association between** hepatoblastoma and Beckwith-Wiedemann syndrome.
   3. **Hepatoblastoma is not related** to pre-existing liver disease, such as cirrhosis (in contrast to hepatocellular carcinoma).
   4. The **pathologic features** include four subtypes
       —fetal.
       —embryonal.
       —macrotrabecular.
       —small-cell undifferentiated.

5. These **tumors**

—may be pedunculated, and **vascular invasion is common.**

—may contain areas of **extramedullary hematopoiesis.**

6. The **clinical presentation**

—is that of a distinct mass in the right upper quadrant.

  a. The **tumor may secrete**

    —**human chorionic gonadotropin (β-HCG)**, leading to isosexual precocity in male patients.

  b. The tumor marker **α-fetoprotein**

    —**is elevated** in over 90% of these tumors and levels should be documented.

7. **Abdominal CT scan or magnetic resonance imaging (MRI)**

—demonstrates the extent of disease and its relationship to vascular structures.

8. **Outcome for patients** with hepatoblastoma

—is largely dependent on resectability, thus, the primary goal of therapy is resection.

  a. **Primary resection is the optimal form of therapy.** Next is by high-dose doxorubicin and cisplatin.

  b. For **initially unresectable tumors, preoperative chemotherapy may allow for later resection of an otherwise unresectable tumor.**

9. **Survival**

—is related to histology and resectability of the tumor.

  a. **Pure fetal histology tumors**

    —that are completely excised have a nearly 90% long-term survival rate.

  b. **Mixed tumors**

    —completely resected, have a long-term survival rate of approximately 60%.

Review Test

Directions: Each of the numbered items or incomplete statements in this section is followed by answers or by completions of the statement. Select the ONE lettered answer or completion that is BEST in each case.

1. A newborn boy is noted to experience a choking episode during the first feeding attempt. The child is noted to have excessive drooling. There is no respiratory distress when the child is not feeding. An orogastric tube does not pass the estimated distance into the stomach, meeting obstruction just past the oropharynx. A chest/abdomen radiograph reveals the orogastric tube to be coiled at the level of the third thoracic vertebra. Lung fields are normal, and the abdomen appears to have a normal distribution of air. Which of the following is the most likely diagnosis?

(A) Acquired esophageal stenosis
(B) Esophageal atresia
(C) Esophageal atresia with proximal fistula
(D) Proximal esophageal atresia with distal tracheoesophageal fistula
(E) Isolated tracheoesophageal fistula

2. A 3-week-old boy is being evaluated for persistent vomiting for the past 4 days. The emesis has been nonbilious and forceful with every feeding. The child is hungry after each episode of emesis. Examination reveals mildly decreased skin turgor, dry mucous membranes, and a nondistended abdomen. There is a palpable pyloric tumor in the midepigastrium. Which of the following is the most likely diagnosis?

(A) Malrotation with midgut volvulus
(B) Duodenal atresia
(C) Annular pancreas
(D) Pyloric stenosis
(E) Jejunal atresia

3. A 2-week-old child is being evaluated in a local emergency room for green-stained vomiting. The mother reports that the child had been well until today, when he began vomiting and developed abdominal distension. The child is awake and crying inconsolably with a distended abdomen. There are no palpable abdominal masses. Intravenous access is established. A plain abdominal radiograph reveals a nonobstructive gas pattern. Among the possible diagnoses listed, which of the following is the most life-threatening condition in the acute period?

(A) Viral gastroenteritis
(B) Lactose intolerance
(C) Malrotation with midgut volvulus
(D) Hirschsprung disease
(E) Pyloric stenosis

4. A newborn child is noted to have a small umbilical defect to the right of a normal-appearing umbilical cord. The bowel is encased in a matted mass of inflammatory tissue. Which of the following is most consistent with these findings?

(A) Gastroschisis
(B) Omphalocele
(C) Umbilical hernia
(D) Diaphragmatic hernia
(E) Prune-belly syndrome

5. A 1-day-old child is referred for evaluation of abdominal distension and feeding intolerance. The child has previously passed meconium. On examination, the child is in no distress, the abdomen is mildly distended, and bowel sounds are normal. An abdominal radiograph shows several air fluid levels in the upper abdomen. There is no air in the distal bowel. Which of the following is the most likely diagnosis?

(A) Duodenal atresia
(B) Jejunal atresia
(C) Hirschsprung disease
(D) Imperforate anus
(E) Esophageal atresia with tracheoesophageal fistula

6. A 2-day-old infant presents in the nursery with persistent bilious emesis since birth. Physical examination reveals a distended abdomen. An upper gastrointestinal series reveals obstruction at the level of the ileum with a stricture approximately 4 cm long. Which of the following is the most likely cause of this anomaly?

(A) Failure of recanalization following a period of mucosal overgrowth
(B) Failure of craniocaudal migration of the myenteric plexus of nerves
(C) Intrauterine vascular compromise resulting in involution of the associated segment of bowel
(D) Intrauterine midgut volvulus
(E) Failure of the midgut to return to the abdominal cavity following the elongation phase of intestinal development

7. A 1-day-old infant with trisomy 21 develops bilious emesis after the first feeding. Which of the following characteristic findings would most likely suggest the diagnosis of duodenal atresia?

(A) String sign on contrast upper gastrointestinal film
(B) Abdominal distension and bilious emesis
(C) Double bubble sign on plain abdominal film
(D) Palpable epigastric mass
(E) Persistent jaundice with a right upper quadrant mass

8. A 1-week-old male infant presents to the emergency room with a 12-hour history of bilious emesis. The parents state that the baby has been crying since the onset of the emesis and that the symptoms developed acutely. Among the choices below, which of the following is the next step in the management of this child?

(A) Resuscitation and stool cultures
(B) Contrast upper gastrointestinal series
(C) Abdominal ultrasound
(D) Resuscitation and rectal biopsy
(E) Obtain blood sample for serum electrolytes

9. A newborn child has an umbilical defect covered by a jelly-like material and umbilical vessels arising from the top of the lesion. Which of the following is the most likely diagnosis?

(A) Gastroschisis
(B) Omphalocele
(C) Umbilical hernia
(D) Diaphragmatic hernia
(E) Prune belly syndrome

10. A woman is referred to your office for prenatal counseling. She is pregnant at 28 weeks gestation and the obstetrician has identified a defect in the left hemidiaphragm. Upon discussion of this condition with the parents, which of the following is an appropriate statement regarding congenital diaphragm hernia (CDH)?

(A) The defect is more common on the right than on the left
(B) CDH is rarely associated with other anomalies
(C) The survival rate for CDH is approximately 60%
(D) The cause of failure in these newborns is related to mediastinal shift caused by the presence of the defect
(E) Operative treatment should be undertaken immediately once the child is born

11. A 6-week-old boy presents to the emergency room with a 3–4 day history of worsening nonbilious emesis according to his parents. The parents state that he has not "kept a meal down" in the last 36 hours. He is noted to be dehydrated. Abdominal examination reveals a nondistended abdomen and a "pyloric tumor." Which of the following is the most likely electrolyte disturbance in this child?

(A) Metabolic acidosis, hypokalemia, hypochloremia
(B) Metabolic alkalosis, hyperkalemia, hyperchloremia
(C) Metabolic alkalosis, hypokalemia, hyperchloremia
(D) Metabolic acidosis, hyperkalemia, hypochloremia
(E) Metabolic alkalosis, hypokalemia, hypochloremia

12. An otherwise healthy 6-month-old female infant presents to the office with a right groin mass noted by her parents. The parents state that the mass has "come and gone" since birth. On examination, there is a smooth reducible mass in the right groin consistent with a right inguinal hernia. Which of the following is the most appropriate treatment strategy for this patient?

(A) No surgery and re-evaluation in 6 months
(B) Emergent hernia repair via the McVay technique
(C) Emergent operative closure of the processus vaginalis
(D) Elective hernia repair via the McVay technique
(E) Elective operative closure of the processus vaginalis

Answers and Explanations

1-D. Esophageal atresia usually presents with excessive drooling in a child who experiences choking with feedings. The orogastric tube typically coils at the level of atresia. The presence of air in the distal gastrointestinal tract demonstrates a distal tracheoesophageal fistula. In the absence of distal fistula, there is no gas on the abdominal radiograph. Isolated fistula occurs without atresia, but is differentiated by the passage of the orogastric tube. Acquired esophageal stenosis does not frequently present in newborns.

2-D. Hypertrophic pyloric stenosis typically occurs at 3 weeks of age and is associated with persistent nonbilious vomiting. Children may become dehydrated as the disease progresses. The palpation of a pyloric tumor is diagnostic of pyloric stenosis. Malrotation, annular pancreas, and jejunal atresia typically present with bilious emesis. Despite the proximal nature of the obstruction, duodenal atresia also typically presents with bilious emesis because the atretic segments are frequently beyond the ampulla of Vater.

3-C. The patient's clinical description is the typical presentation of malrotation with midgut volvulus. Viral gastroenteritis may present with emesis but frequently presents with diarrhea as well. The suspicion of pyloric stenosis is based on history and is not likely in the patient presented because these children usually do not have bilious emesis or abdominal distension. Hirschsprung disease is usually suspected on the basis of delayed passage of meconium in the newborn period. Formula- or lactose-intolerance is not usually associated with bilious emesis.

4-A. Gastroschisis is usually a small umbilical defect through which the bowel herniates. There is no covering sac, and the bowel therefore becomes encased in an inflammatory process. Unless ruptured, an omphalocele is generally covered by mesenchyma (Wharton's jelly). An umbilical hernia is covered by skin. A diaphragmatic hernia does not present as an umbilical defect. Prune belly syndrome is a congenital absence of abdominal wall musculature and is not associated with exposed bowel.

5-B. Jejunal atresia presents in the newborn period with feeding intolerance and abdominal distension related to the level of atresia. These children are not usually in distress, although massive abdominal distension may lead to respiratory distress. Duodenal atresia is not associated with dilated loops of small bowel or with distal air fluid levels. Hirschsprung disease is associated with delayed passage of meconium and massive abdominal distension. Imperforate anus is diagnosed by the physical finding of absent or abnormally located anus. In esophageal atresia, there is an absence of stomach air.

6-C. This patient's findings are consistent with ileal atresia. Small bowel atresias are the result of an intrauterine vascular event leading to ischemic involution of the associated portion of bowel. The other descriptions given are not causes of primary congenital intestinal atresia.

7-C. Duodenal atresia is classically diagnosed by the finding of a double bubble sign on plain abdominal radiograph, usually with little or no distal gas. Upper gastrointestinal film may confirm the double bubble, but string sign is more indicative of pyloric stenosis than duodenal atresia. These children do not have abdominal distension, because the level of obstruction does not permit gas to pass into the distal bowel. A palpable epigastric or right upper quadrant mass is not associated with duodenal atresia.

8-B. All children presenting with bilious emesis should be suspected of having a surgical problem until proven otherwise. The upper gastrointestinal series is the most reliable diagnostic study to rule out malrotation. The diagnostic upper gastrointestinal series in the child suspected of having midgut volvulus should be obtained immediately, because the delayed diagnosis is nearly uniformly fatal.

9-B. Omphalocele is an umbilical defect covered by mesenchyma (Wharton's jelly). The umbilical vessels insert into the top of the sac. Omphalocele is associated with a 35%–80% incidence of other anomalies, many lethal. Gastroschisis is usually an isolated defect, although it may be associated with intestinal atresia. An umbilical hernia is covered by skin. A diaphragmatic hernia does not present as an umbilical defect. Prune belly syndrome is a congenital absence of abdominal wall musculature and is not associated with exposed bowel.

10-C. Congenital diaphragm hernia (CDH) results from a failure of fusion of the pleuroperitoneal membrane during the eighth week of gestation. It occurs most commonly on the left side in the posterolateral position (foramen of Bochdalek). Approximately 50% of these children have associated anomalies, most commonly cardiac or neural tube defects. The diagnosis is frequently made by prenatal ultrasound, and overall survival is approximately 60%. These patients usually present with respiratory distress as a result of both pulmonary hypoplasia and pulmonary hypertension. Mediastinal shift is not a significant contributor to the initial respiratory compromise. Operative therapy does not improve the respiratory function of the child, because it does nothing to address the pulmonary hypoplasia or hypertension. Operative intervention, therefore, should be delayed until the child is stable.

11-E. Children with pyloric stenosis develop volume depletion as a result of inadequate enteral absorption of feedings. The typical electrolyte disturbance of metabolic alkalosis, with hypokalemia and hypochloremia, develops from both gastrointestinal and renal causes. The child vomits against a closed pylorus, resulting in a loss of hydrogen and chloride ions found in gastric secretions. As the child becomes volume depleted, aldosterone-mediated resorption of sodium ions in the distal tubule leads to further renal loss of hydrogen and potassium ions. The result of these losses is paradoxical aciduria and contraction alkalosis.

12-E. Inguinal hernias in infants are the result of a persistent patent processus vaginalis communicating with the peritoneal cavity. These hernias are thus indirect hernias rather than direct. Appropriate treatment in this setting involves elective operative closure of the processus vaginalis at the earliest convenient time without the need for formal fascial closure, as in adults. Similar to adults, emergent operative repair is indicated for nonreducible or strangulated hernias, but is not necessary in an uncomplicated reducible hernia.

4

Otolaryngology

David Dorofi

I. Anatomy

A. Characteristics of the cranial nerves

—are outlined in **Table 4-1.**

1. An **understanding of these characteristics**

   —is essential in the diagnosis and treatment of disorders of the head and neck.

2. **CN V, VII, IX, and X**

   —all have sensory components for the ear, which are also important for referred pain from the mouth and pharynx.

B. Bony components of the skull

1. The **orbit** consists of **7 bones**

   —frontal.

   —zygomatic.

   —sphenoid.

   —ethmoid.

   —lacrimal.

   —maxilla.

   —palatine.

2. The **sella turcica** is a depression in the sphenoid bone that houses the pituitary gland.

3. The **paranasal sinuses** include the paired maxillary sinuses, anterior and posterior ethmoid, and the sphenoid sinuses.

   —The paranasal sinuses are lined by **modified ciliated respiratory epithelium,** which produce approximately 1.5 L of mucus a day.

93

Table 4-1. The Cranial Nerves

Number	Name	Sensation	Motor	Parasympathetic
I	**Olfactory**	Smell		
II	**Optic**	Sight		
III	**Oculomotor**		Superior, medial, inferior rectus, inferior oblique, levator palpebrae superioris muscles	Constrictor pupillae and ciliary muscles
IV	**Trochlear**		**Superior oblique muscle (SO$_4$)**	
V	**Trigeminal** **V$_1$**: ophthalmic branch **V$_2$**: maxillary branch **V$_3$**: mandibular branch	**V$_1$**: conjunctiva, cornea, eye, orbit, forehead and face, sinuses **V$_2$**: nasal cavity, palate, nasopharynx **V$_3$**: oral cavity, mandible, anterior neck	**V$_3$**: muscles of mastication **(masseter, temporalis, medial** and **lateral pterygoid), tensor tympani** (connected to malleus bone) and **tensor veli palatini** muscles	
VI	**Abducens**		**Lateral rectus** muscle **(LR$_6$)**	
VII	**Facial**	Taste to the **anterior ⅔ of tongue**	Muscles of **facial expression, posterior belly of digastric, stylohyoid, stapedius**	Submandibular and sublingual glands via the chorda tympani nerve and lingual nerve, lacrimal gland
VIII	**Vestibulocochlear**	**Cochlea** (hearing) and **semicircular canals** (vestibular and acceleration sensation)		
IX	**Glossopharyngeal**	Taste to the **posterior ⅓ of tongue**, ear (Jacobson's nerve)	**Stylopharyngeus** and **superior pharyngeal constrictor** muscles	**Parotid gland** via the lesser superficial petrosal nerve, carotid body and sinus
X	**Vagus**	Ear (Arnold's nerve)	Palatoglossus, middle and inferior pharyngeal constrictor, levator veli palatini muscles, smooth muscles of the thoracic and abdominal viscera, muscles of the larynx (vocal cords)	Gastrointestinal tract
XI	**Accessory**		**Sternocleidomastoid** (SCM) and **trapezius** muscles	
XII	**Hypoglossal**		Intrinsic muscles of the **tongue**	

C. **Upper respiratory tract (Figure 4.1)**

1. The **roof** of the **nasal cavity**

    —houses the cribriform plate with the olfactory epithelium (CN I).

    a. **Three turbinates**

    —(inferior, middle, superior) arise from the lateral wall with a meatus or opening under each turbinate.

    b. The **ethmoid sinuses**

    —(frontal, maxillary, and anterior) drain into the middle meatus.

    c. The **posterior ethmoid and sphenoid sinuses**

    —drain into the superior meatus.

    d. The **nasal lacrimal duct**

    —that drains tears empties into the inferior meatus.

2. The **nasopharynx**

    —is below the sphenoid sinuses.

    —contains the **adenoid tonsils** (posterior) and the **torus tubarius** with the opening of the **eustachian tube.**

3. The **oropharynx** contains the

    —soft palate.

    —base of the tongue.

    —tonsillar pillars.

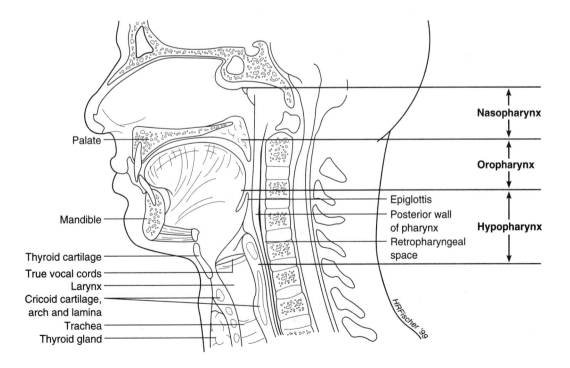

Figure 4.1. Sagittal section of upper respiratory tract and pharynx. (Adapted with permission from Agur AMR, Lee, MJ: *Grant's Atlas of Anatomy,* 9th ed. Baltimore, Williams & Wilkins, 1991, p 605.)

—**palatine tonsils.**

—**vallecula** (area between the epiglottis and base of tongue).

4. The **larynx (Figure 4.2)**

a. The **true vocal cords (glottis)**

—include the vocalis muscles that are innervated by the **superior and recurrent laryngeal nerves** (CN X).

(1) The superior laryngeal nerve innervates the **cricothyroid muscle.**

(2) All other intrinsic laryngeal muscles are innervated by the recurrent laryngeal nerve.

b. The **false cords**

—are superior to the true cords.

5. The **trachea**

—begins at the cricoid (C5–6) and ends at the carina (T4–6).

a. The **anterior and lateral walls** contain U-shaped cartilage rings.

b. The **posterior wall** or membranous portion is made up of a muscular layer.

c. The **blood supply** in the neck is from the inferior thyroid vessels.

D. **Triangles of the neck**

1. The **anterior triangle**

a. is **bound by** the

—anterior border of the sternocleidomastoid (SCM).

—sternal notch.

—inferior border of digastrics.

b. contains the **carotid sheath.**

2. The **posterior triangle**

a. is **bound by** the

—posterior border of the SCM.

—trapezius muscle.

—clavicle.

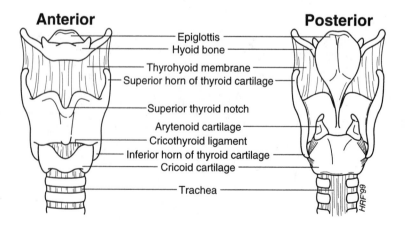

Figure 4.2. The larynx.

b. **contains CN XI** and the **brachial plexus.**

E. **Salivary glands**

1. **These exocrine glands** consist of

—the large paired **parotid, submandibular,** and **sublingual glands** and numerous minor glands.

2. The **parotid glands (Figure 4.3)**

—are the largest salivary glands.

—are located lateral to the angle of the mandible.

—**Stensen's duct** empties the saliva from the parotids at the second upper molar.

3. The **submandibular glands**

—are located medial and inferior to the body/angle of the mandible as they wrap around the mylohyoid muscle.

—**Wharton's duct** empties the saliva from these glands into the anterior floor of the mouth.

4. The **sublingual glands**

—are the smallest of the large salivary glands.

—are located beneath the anterior tongue.

—These glands empty into small **ducts of Rivinus** in the anterior floor of the mouth.

5. The **minor salivary glands**

—are located throughout the oral cavity and oropharynx and number between 700–1000.

F. **Ear (Figure 4.4)**

1. The **ear is divided** into three portions

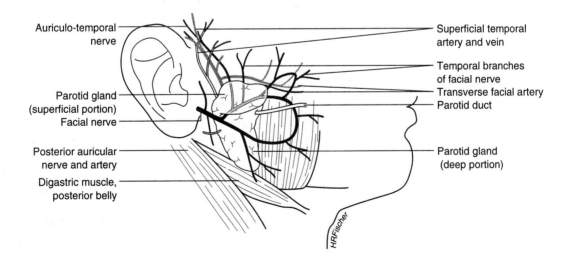

Figure 4.3. The parotid gland. (Adapted with permission from Agur AMR, Lee, MJ: *Grant's Atlas of Anatomy,* 9th ed. Baltimore, Williams & Wilkins, 1991, p 494.)

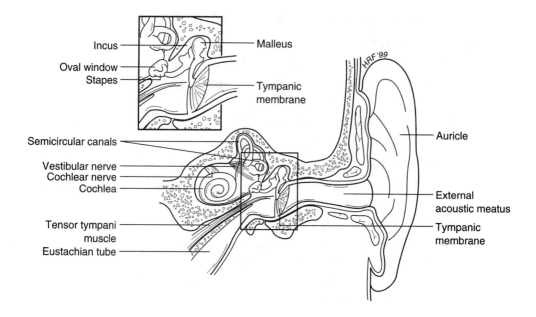

Figure 4.4. Structures of the ear.

—**external.**

—**middle.**

—**inner.**

2. The **external ear** is comprised of the

—auricle.

—external auditory canal.

3. The **middle ear**

   a. The middle ear is **comprised** of the

      —tympanic membrane (TM).

      —**three ossicles** (malleus, incus, stapes).

      —eustachian tube.

   b. It is **connected to** the mastoid air cells.

   c. The **stapes** articulates with the **oval window** of the inner ear.

4. The **inner ear**

   a. The inner ear **consists** of the

      —**cochlea.**

      —**labyrinth** (three semicircular canals).

      —internal auditory canal.

   b. The **semicircular canals** include the

      —**superior** (anterior) canals.

      —**horizontal** (lateral) canals.

      —**posterior canals.**

   c. The **vestibular division of CN VIII**

—innervates the canals.

5. The **cochlea**

   a. **contains** the hearing organ or **Corti's organ.**

      —Corti's organ is lined with **inner and outer hair** cells.

      (1) The **inner hair** cells transmit sound impulse (**afferent**).

      (2) The **outer hair** cells receive **efferent** impulses from the central nervous system.

   b. The **cochlea is innervated** by the **cochlear division of CN VIII.**

G. Blood supply

   1. The **main blood supply** of the head and neck is from the **internal** and **external carotid arteries** and the **thyrocervical trunk.**

   2. The **internal carotid artery** has no branches in the neck.

      —The **ophthalmic artery,** an intracranial branch, traverses the orbit and forms the **supratrochlear** and **supraorbital** arteries to supply the forehead.

   3. The **major branches** of the **external carotid artery include the following arteries:**

      —superior thyroid.

      —ascending pharyngeal.

      —lingual.

      —facial.

      —occipital.

      —posterior auricular.

      —maxillary.

      —superficial temporal.

   4. The **thyrocervical trunk** supplies many structures in the lower neck.

   5. The **veins accompany the arteries** and empty into the **external** and **internal jugular veins.**

   6. Epistaxis

      —is bleeding from the nose, most commonly (90%) from the anterior septum in an area called **Little's area** (Kiesselbach's plexus).

H. Lymphatics

   1. The skin and subcutaneous tissues of the face and scalp drain into the local lymphatics.

      a. The **temporal areas**

         —drain into the pre-auricular and **parotid** lymph nodes.

      b. The **occipital region**

         —drains into the **posterior neck** nodes.

      c. The **parotid gland**

         —drains into the intra-parotid nodes and **anterior cervical** (jugulodigastric) nodes.

d. The **nasal cavity**

—drains into the retropharyngeal and deep cervical nodes.

e. The **nasopharynx**

—drains into the retropharyngeal, jugulodigastric, and deep cervical nodes.

2. The **anterior floor of the mouth,** the tongue, and the lower lips

—drain bilaterally into the **submandibular nodes.**

3. The **buccal mucosa**

—drains into the ipsilateral submandibular nodes.

4. The **hard palate**

—drains into the upper cervical nodes.

5. The **oropharynx** and the **base of the tongue**

—have **bilateral** drainage into the deep cervical nodes.

6. The **soft palate**

—drains into the **retropharyngeal** nodes.

7. The **larynx** and **hypopharynx**

—drain into **the cervical nodes.**

8. The **epiglottis**

—has **bilateral** drainage into the deep cervical nodes.

II. Physiology

A. Swallowing

—consists of three phases: **oral, pharyngeal, esophageal.**

1. The **oral phase**

—is voluntary.

—consists of bolus control and delivery.

2. The **pharyngeal phase**

—is involuntary.

—starts when the bolus enters the oropharynx until it passes into the esophagus.

3. The **esophageal phase**

—consists of involuntary peristalsis.

B. Laryngeal functions

1. The **larynx serves three functions:**

—speech.

—airway protection.

—respiration.

2. **Speech**

—is created when the true vocal cords **adduct** and vibrate.

3. A **patient may have a normal voice**

—if the **vocal cords are paralyzed** in an adducted position, but the patient will have a compromised airway.

4. During **respiration** the cords **abduct.**

C. **Salivary glands**

1. **Saliva contains**

—serous fluid with electrolytes (low Na^+, high K^+).

—immunoglobulin (Ig) A.

—amylase.

—mucin.

—enzymes.

—Saliva has a basic pH.

2. **Gland secretion**

—The **parotid glands secrete** mostly **serous** fluid.

—The **sublingual glands** secrete mostly **mucin.**

—The **submandibular glands** are 50/50.

3. Between **500–1500 mL** of saliva is produced each day.

4. **Activation**

—**Sympathetic** activation inhibits secretion.

—**Parasympathetic** activation stimulates secretion.

D. **Hearing and balance**

1. **When sound waves strike the TM,** the ossicular chain waves are created in cochlear fluid.

—This moves the basilar membrane and vibrates and triggers the **inner hair cells.**

2. The **basilar membrane**

—widens toward the apex of the cochlea so **lower frequency sounds** are heard at the **apex** and higher frequency sounds are heard at the base.

3. **Sensorineural hearing** refers to **CN VIII** and the **cochlea.**

—**Conductive hearing** refers to the **TM** and **ossicular chain.**

4. The **TM** and the **ossicles**

—**increase** the sound energy by **17:1.**

5. **Acceleration**

—**Hair cells located** in the semicircular canals **are responsible for** rotational acceleration.

—The **macula,** located in the **utricle,** and **saccule** transmit **gravitational** and **linear acceleration signals.**

III. Infections of the Head and Neck (Table 4-2)

A. Upper respiratory tract

1. **Rhinitis**

    —is an inflammation of the nasal mucosa caused by viruses (e.g., rhinovirus).

    a. Symptoms are nasal congestion and drainage.

    b. Treat only symptomatically.

2. **Rhinitis medicamentosa**

    —is a syndrome of nasal congestion seen with the long-term **abuse of decongestant sprays** (e.g., sympathomimetics).

3. **Allergic rhinitis**

    —is caused by environmental allergens (e.g., pollen).

    —is associated with elevated serum **IgE** and nasal mucous **eosinophilia.**

    —Treat symptomatically or with desensitization immunotherapy (allergy shots).

B. Sinusitis (see Table 4-2)

1. **Acute sinusitis**

    a. **Risk factors** include

       —allergy.

       —nasal polyposis.

       —**obstructive foreign bodies (e.g., nasogastric tube).**

       —upper respiratory infections.

       —maxillary dental infections.

    b. **Computed tomography (CT) scan**

       —is reserved for recurrent acute sinusitis.

       —characteristically demonstrates air fluid levels within the sinus.

2. **Chronic sinusitis**

    —is characterized by persistent bacterial infection lasting longer than 4–6 weeks or recurrent infections.

    a. **Treatment** involves

       —administering long-term antibiotics.

       —functional endoscopic sinus surgery (FESS) if antibiotics fail.

    b. **FESS**

       —involves clearing the sinus ostium to allow for unobstructed **normal ciliary clearance** of the sinuses.

       —is indicated for anatomical obstructions of the sinus ostium, chronic sinusitis, severe nasal polyposis, or severe chronic diseases (e.g., cystic fibrosis).

C. Tonsillitis (see Table 4-2)

1. **Tonsillar tissue** consists of

Table 4-2. Head and Neck Infections

Infection	Site	Signs and Symptoms	Organisms	Treatment
Sinusitis	Sinus	Low-grade fever, malaise, facial pain, anterior nasal discharge, postnasal drip	Acute: *Streptococcus pneumoniae, Staphylococcus aureus, Streptococcus pyogenes* Chronic: anaerobic organisms (*Bacteroides* species) or *S. aureus, Haemophilus influenzae,* streptococci	Antibiotics, decongestants, nasal hygiene, removal of foreign bodies (e.g., NG tubes), FESS occasionally used for chronic disease
Tonsillitis	Palatine tonsils	Enlarged tonsils, cervical adenopathy, tonsillar exudate; exudate, malaise and adenopathy may suggest mononucleosis	Viral: adenovirus, enterovirus, coxsackievirus; mononucleosis caused by Epstein-Barr virus; mixed oropharyngeal flora	Antibiotics for bacterial disease (if untreated, a peritonsillar abscess may develop that requires incision and drainage); tonsillectomy indicated for recurrent disease
Epiglottitis	Supraglottis	Airway obstruction, high fever, stridor, severe throat pain mainly in children (ages 3–5)	*Haemophilus influenzae* type B	Antibiotics, early airway control if necessary
Croup (larngotracheal bronchitis)	Subglottis	Sudden onset, characteristic barking cough mainly in children (6 months to 3 years old)	Parainfluenza virus	Airway monitoring, humidified air, racemic epinephrine
Pharyngitis	Pharynx	Sore throat, fever, enlarged tonsils, cervical adenopathy, exudate only in 50% of bacterial infections	Viral: adenovirus, enterovirus, coxsackievirus Bacterial: Group A β-hemolytic streptococci	Antibiotics for bacterial disease, untreated disease may lead to rheumatic fever or acute glomerulonephritis
Deep neck abscess	Deep neck space	Fever, elevated WBC, neck swelling, possible airway obstruction, mediastinitis	*S. aureus, S. pyogenes, Peptostreptococcus, Bacteroides* species, *Fusobacterium*	Surgical drainage, antibiotics, airway monitoring

(continued)

Table 4-2. Head and Neck Infections

Infection	Site	Signs and Symptoms	Organisms	Treatment
Parotitis	Parotid	Unilateral parotid swelling and pain, overlying erythema, purulence from Stensen's duct; often associated with dehydration	*S. aureus,* gram-negative rods in critically ill patients	Warm compresses, antibiotics, fluids, and sialogogues (lemon drops)
Otitis media	Middle ear	Ear ache, fever, middle ear effusion, bulging tympanic membrane, conductive hearing loss if chronic	*S. pneumoniae, H. influenza, Moraxella catarrhalis*	Antibiotics, rarely myringotomy, pressure equalization tubes for chronic disease
Otitis externa (swimmer's ear)	Ear canal	Extreme ear pain and some times ear drainage	*Pseudomonas* species followed by *Staphylococcus* species	Acidic ear drops, oral antibiotics, pain control, and dry ear precautions
Labyrinthitis	Inner ear	Vertigo, nystagmus, nausea, vomiting; hearing loss and fever may be associated with suppurative infection	Frequently viral; suppurative (bacterial) infection associated with same organisms as middle ear	Supportive therapy for viral disease; intravenous antibiotics for suppurative disease

NG = nasogastric; FESS = functional endoscopic sinus surgery; WBC = white blood cells.

—the palatine.

—adenoids tonsils.

2. A **peritonsillar abscess**

—may result from an untreated pharyngitis.

a. The **abscess forms** between the tonsil and the lateral pharyngeal wall.

b. **Treat** with incision and drainage, along with antibiotics.

D. **Epiglottitis** (see Table 4-2)

1. **Affected children** classically are found

—leaning forward in the sitting position.

—drooling.

—with severe respiratory stridor.

2. The **classic radiographic finding** is the **thumbprint sign** on a lateral neck film caused by epiglottic swelling.

—This **finding is rarely seen** because of widespread immunization with the *Haemophilus influenzae* type B **(Hib) vaccine.**

3. **Treatment**

—involves early **airway control** with intubation or tracheostomy and antibiotics.

E. **Infections of the deep neck spaces**

1. The **fascial layers of the head and neck** are potential areas for spread of infections.

2. These **fascial layers include** the **superficial cervical fascia** and the **deep cervical fascia** that is further divided into the superficial, middle, and deep layers.

—All three layers of the deep cervical fascia form the **carotid sheath** that extends from the skull base to the mediastinum.

3. **Deep neck space infections**

—form from complications of pharyngitis, dental caries, and trauma.

—have the **potential to spread** throughout the head and neck via the potential spaces created by the **fascial planes.**

F. **Ludwig's angina**

—is an acute infection of the floor of the mouth that invades the mylohyoid muscle.

1. The **most common primary cause** is **dental infection** of the mandibular teeth.

2. This **may rapidly spread** to deeper neck spaces and may cause **airway obstruction.**

3. **Treatment** involves **airway control** by tracheostomy or intubation.

—Surgical drainage and antibiotics follow.

G. **Sialoadenitis**

—is an acute infection of a salivary gland and is often caused by **sialolithiasis** (stones in the duct).

1. The **submandibular gland** is affected 80% of the time.

2. **Treatment** involves

—application of warm compresses.

—antibiotics.

—fluid administration.

—sialogogues.

—stone removal, if possible.

H. **Infections of the ear**

1. **Otitis media** (OM) (see Table 4-2)

—is an infection of the middle ear.

—may be categorized as **acute suppurative, chronic serous,** or **chronic suppurative.**

a. **Acute suppurative OM**

—is a **bacterial** infection that often follows a viral upper respiratory tract infection.

(1) This is characterized by **purulent** middle ear fluid with bulging TMs.

(2) The major offenders are *Streptococcus pneumoniae, H. influenza,* and *Moraxella catarrhalis.*

(3) Treat with **antibiotics,** although myringotomy (incision in TM) may be necessary in some situations.

b. **Chronic serous OM**

—is characterized by a persistent serous middle ear effusion.

(1) **Eustachian tube dysfunction** is most often implicated as the cause.

(2) This is very common in **children** and may lead to speech delay secondary to long-term conductive hearing loss.

(3) **Pressure equalization tubes** (PE tubes) placed across the TM are often required for treatment.

c. **Chronic suppurative OM**

—implies a persistent TM perforation with drainage more common in patients with chronic ear disease.

(1) This is most commonly caused by *Pseudomonas aeruginosa.*

(2) With recurrent disease, care must be taken to rule out potential causes (e.g., tumors, eustachian tube dysfunction, allergies).

(3) **Treatment** is the same as with otitis externa (see Table 4-2).

(4) **Tympanoplasty** (perforation repair) may be required.

2. **Necrotizing otitis externa**

—or skull base osteomyelitis is an extremely **severe infection** of the skull base.

a. This is usually caused by *P. aeruginosa.*

b. This infection is **most commonly seen** in elderly patients with poorly controlled diabetes or immunocompromised patients.

c. **Treatment** involves long-term, high-dose antibiotic therapy.

3. **Coalescent mastoiditis**

—is an infection of the mastoid air cells with a mastoid abscess and destruction of bone.

a. **Although rare, this generally results as** a complication of untreated acute suppurative OM.

b. **Patients present with**

—**fevers.**

—high white blood cell count.

—a pushed forward ear.

—**fluctuant,** swelling, and erythema over the mastoid.

c. To **prevent serious complications,** this **severe form of mastoiditis requires**

—**emergent treatment** with surgical **mastoidectomy.**

—intravenous (IV) antibiotics.

d. **Complications** may include

—sigmoid sinus thrombosis.

—meningitis.

—brain abscess.

—facial nerve injury.

—death.

4. Bell's palsy

—is an acute paralysis of **CN VII.**

—is the most common cause of **facial paralysis.**

a. Patients are often asymptomatic

—except for some occasional otalgia (ear pain, 20%) and taste complaints via the chorda tympani nerve.

b. The **peak incidence**

—occurs between the age of **20–40 years.**

c. The **etiology**

—is thought to be related to **herpes simplex virus** infection.

d. Complete paralysis may develop within 48 hours, and resolution may take several months.

—If the paralysis does not resolve within 6 months, other potential causes should be evaluated (i.e., tumor).

e. Treatment

—may involve steroid therapy and possibly antiviral agents.

5. Herpes zoster oticus (Ramsay Hunt's syndrome)

—is an infection of **CN VII.**

a. Symptoms may include

—otalgia.

—facial paralysis.

—**herpes vesicles** in the external auditory canal and on the face.

b. Treatment

—is the same as for Bell's palsy (see III H 4 e).

6. Sudden sensorineural hearing loss

—is the acute onset of severe hearing loss with no obvious cause.

a. A **viral etiology** has been suggested.

b. Ninety percent of the time, this occurs unilaterally.

c. Factors associated with a good recovery

—include minimal low-frequency hearing loss and a young age.

d. Treatment

—involves steroid therapy and possibly antiviral agents.

IV. Neoplasms of the Head and Neck (Table 4-4)

A. Cutaneous malignancies

—are the most common cancers of the head and neck.

—are related to sun exposure (see *BRS General Surgery,* Chapter 21 II A).

Table 4-4. Head and Neck Neoplasms

Site	Neoplasm	Epidemiology	Risk Factors	Signs and Symptoms	Diagnosis	Treatment
Lesions of the skin	Basal cell carcinoma	Elderly Caucasians, common	Sun exposure	Nonhealing lesion; these lesions are slow growing and seldom metastasize	Biopsy	Moh's surgery or excision
	Squamous cell carcinoma (SCCA)	Elderly Caucasians, fairly common	Sun exposure	Nonhealing lesion	Biopsy	Wide excision, possible neck dissection for metastatic nodes, +/− XRT
	Melanoma	Caucasians' risk increase with age but may affect young	Sun exposure but not always	Dark irregular lesion	Punch biopsy	Wide excision, **controversial neck dissection** for metastatic nodes, possible chemotherapy, XRT, and/or immunotherapy.
Paranasal sinus (⅔ occur in the maxillary sinus)	Squamous cell carcinoma (80%)	Elderly, rare	Woodworkers, metal refiners, textile workers, and nickel workers	Nasal obstruction, epistaxis, sinusitis	Biopsy	Wide excision, possible neck dissection for metastatic nodes, may require adjuvant XRT; survival for early stages >70%
	Adenocarcinoma (15%)	Elderly, very rare	Same as SCCA	Nasal obstruction, epistaxis, sinusitis	Biopsy	Same as SCCA
	Esthesioneuroblastoma (rare tumor of olfactory neuroepithelium)	Elderly, very rare	Unknown	Nasal obstruction, epistaxis, sinusitis	Biopsy	Same as SCCA, preoperative chemoradiation therapy may be useful; poor survival
	Juvenile nasopharyngeal angiofibroma	Young adolescent males	Unknown	Nasal obstruction, intermittent epistaxis	CT scan, biopsy not required	Preoperative embolization followed by surgical excision

Lesions of the oral cavity, pharynx, and larynx	SCCA	Elderly, M>F	Tobacco and alcohol abuse	Leukoplakia, chronic sore throat, hoarseness, neck mass, otalgia, stridor	Laryngoscopy with biopsy	Treatment depends on the stage and varies greatly; any combination of surgery, XRT, chemotherapy
Salivary gland (SG) lesions	Pleomorphic adenoma (benign mixed tumor)	M = F, middle age, 80% parotid, accounts for ⅔ of all salivary gland neoplasms	XRT but most not	Painless mass; 1% rate of malignant degeneration (carcinoma expleomorphic)	FNA	Surgical excision via superficial parotidectomy with sparing of the facial nerve
	Warthin's tumor (papillary cystadenoma lymphomatosum)	M:F, 5:1, middle age; benign slow growing tumor accounting for 10% of neoplasms	Unknown	Painless mass, 10% bilateral	FNA	Surgical excision, superficial parotidectomy
	Mucoepidermoid carcinoma	Middle age, 70% parotid, most common malignancy of SG	XRT but most not	Painful mass (13%), facial nerve paralysis, lymphadenopathy	FNA	Surgical excision; total parotidectomy (including facial nerve) with postoperative radiation therapy for intermediate and high grade lesions
	Adenoid cystic carcinoma	Middle age; submandibular gland most commonly involved	Unknown	Painful mass, 20% with facial pain and CN VII invasion	FNA	Surgical excision, total parotidectomy, possible CN VII excision

XRT = x-ray therapy; CT = computed tomography; M = male; F = female; FNA = fine needle aspiration; CN = cranial nerve.

1. Basal cell carcinoma

—is the least aggressive.

—is the most common tumor, accounting for **90% of skin cancers** in the head and neck.

2. Squamous cell carcinoma

—is generally more aggressive.

—accounts for **10% of skin cancers.**

a. Their **metastatic potential** depends on the depth of invasion.

b. These lesions may **frequently spread** to local lymph nodes.

3. Melanoma

—is the most aggressive cutaneous malignancy.

a. **Survival and metastatic potential**

—are directly related to the depth of invasion or the thickness of the tumor (see *BRS General Surgery,* Chapter 21 I D 1).

b. **Delayed metastatic disease**

—is not uncommon, so long-term follow-up is essential.

B. Solid malignancies of the upper respiratory tract

—are **staged** by the **TNM classification system** (see *BRS General Surgery,* Chapter 21, Table 21-1).

C. Lesions of the oral cavity, pharynx, and larynx

1. Torus palatini and torus mandibulare

—are common benign bony growths that occur in the oral cavity.

—are often located on the **midline hard palate** and anterior lingual surface of the mandible.

2. Squamous cell carcinoma (see Table 4-3)

—is by far the most common malignancy found in these areas, accounting for greater than **90%** of tumors.

a. **Risk factors** include

—**alcohol** and **tobacco** abuse (including smokeless), which may act synergistically to dramatically increase the risk.

b. **Common sites** include the

—anterior floor or mouth.

—posterior lateral tongue.

—base of the tongue.

—supraglottis (epiglottis).

—glottis (larynx).

(1) **Leukoplakia (white patch) in the oropharynx**

—is frequently a normal finding.

—may be associated with malignancy in high-risk patients (i.e., smokers).

(2) **Tumors of the larynx** may be associated with

—**hoarseness** (most common).

—dyspnea.

—hemoptysis.

—dysphagia.

—weight loss.

c. The overall **5-year survival**

—is **about 50%,** although patients frequently present with late-stage disease (35% 5-year survival).

d. Metastatic spread

—is via lymphatics to the regional drainage pathways.

e. Common sites of distant metastasis include

—lung.

—bone.

—liver.

f. Treatment

—includes a **combination** of surgery, radiation, and chemotherapy with nodal metastases often requiring **neck dissection.**

(1) Neck dissection

—is indicated when there is positive metastatic disease in the neck or when the risk of metastatic disease is high (>70%).

—may either be radical or modified radical.

(2) A **modified radical neck dissection preserves** one or all of the following:

—**internal jugular vein.**

—**SCM muscle.**

—**CN XI.**

3. Benign vocal cord nodules

—may also cause hoarseness in adults.

—are frequently the **result of voice abuse.**

a. These lesions are **characterized by**

—**epithelial hyperplasia.**

—connective tissue fibrosis.

b. Treatment involves

—voice therapy.

—cessation of smoking.

—surgical excision if necessary.

4. Sinonasal undifferentiated carcinoma (SNUC)

—is a very aggressive anaplastic neoplasm of the nasal cavity.

a. This **usually presents** with nasal obstruction and has a very **poor** prognosis.

b. Treatment

—includes chemoradiation, followed by wide local excision.

5. A **neck mass found in a patient**

—with risk factors of tobacco and alcohol abuse is **metastatic cancer** until proven otherwise.

   a. Evaluation should include
   —a full head and neck examination.
   —CT scan.
   —fine needle aspiration (FNA) for diagnosis.
   b. An **excisional biopsy** *should not* be performed.

D. Salivary gland tumors (see Table 4-3)

—occur most commonly in the **parotid gland (80%).**

—are usually benign.

   1. The **risk of malignancy**
   —is generally higher with lesions in the smaller glands.
   a. For example, 5% of salivary neoplasms occur in minor salivary glands, but 80% of those are malignant.
   b. Unlike in adults, the most common salivary gland tumors in children are hemangiomas.
   2. Signs of parotid gland tumors may include
   —facial nerve paralysis.
   —lymphadenopathy.
   —pain (often suggestive of a malignancy).

E. Lesions of the ear
   1. Malignancies of the external and middle ear are rare, but may include squamous cell carcinoma and rhabdomyosarcoma.
   —Nonhealing wounds in this area should be biopsied.
   2. A **cholesteatoma**
   —is an epidermal inclusion cyst located in the middle ear or mastoid.
   a. These **lesions**
      —may be congenital or acquired.
      —are **slow growing,** but will erode as they grow.
   b. The **etiology**
      —may be related to **eustachian tube dysfunction,** with middle ear negative pressure and retracted TM that allows for epidermal ingrowth.
   c. Patients usually present with
      —conductive hearing loss.
      —**chronic draining ear.**
   d. Treatment involves surgical excision.
   3. Acoustic neuromas
   —are schwannomas of CN VIII.
   a. These **lesions most often present** in middle age with symptoms of
      —unilateral progressive hearing loss.
      —tinnitus.
      —dizziness (80%).

    b. Diagnosis is made by
      —T1 contrast-enhanced magnetic resonance imaging (MRI) scan demonstrating a lesion in the internal acoustic canal and/or cerebellopontine angle.

    c. Treatment
      —**Small asymptomatic tumors** in elderly patients may be treated by observation alone.
      —**Surgical excision** is indicated for larger tumors in younger patients and gamma knife radiation as an alternative to surgery (see Chapter 7 II I).

V. Other Types of Ear Disease

A. Otosclerosis

—is a **genetic disease** of the **stapes** footplate.

1. This **disease leads to**
    —an abnormal spongy and sclerotic bone that fixes the footplate, causing a **conductive hearing loss.**

2. Surgical removal of the stapes
    —with prosthetic replacement restores hearing (**stapedectomy**).

B. Ménière's disease

—is a pathological process in the labyrinth and cochlea.

1. This process leads to
    —fluctuating **hearing loss.**
    —**episodic vertigo.**
    —**tinnitus.**
    —aural fullness.

2. The **characteristic histologic finding**
    —is **endolymphatic hydrops** with overexpansion of the endolymphatic spaces.

3. Treatment consists of
    —**low-salt diet.**
    —**diuretics.**
    —antinausea medication.
    —**Surgery** is reserved for refractory cases.

VI. Pediatric Otolaryngology

A. Laryngomalacia

—is the **most common** cause of airway obstruction in infants.

1. Patients frequently present with

—intermittent respiratory distress.

—stridor, exacerbated in the supine position.

2. It is **caused by immature epiglottic cartilage** framework with pro-lapse of the epiglottis over the airway.

3. **Most children grow out** of this by 12 months of age.

—Surgical tracheostomy is reserved for only a small number of the most severe cases.

B. Choanal atresia

—is obstruction of the choanal opening by either bone (90%) or nasal mu-cous membranes.

1. **Affected infants present** with

—intermittent respiratory distress.

—poor suckling during feeds.

2. This obstruction is **usually unilateral.**

3. Because newborns are **obligate nasal breathers,** surgical correction is indicated.

C. Recurrent respiratory papillomatosis

—are the most common tumors of the pediatric larynx.

1. **Patients generally present** with **hoarseness** or respiratory distress.

2. **Papilloma viruses are believed to infect** the larynx after exposure during passage through the birth canal of infected mothers.

3. These **lesions frequently involute** after puberty.

4. **Treatment**

—involves surgical or **laser excision,** although recurrence is common.

D. Cleft lip and palate

—are the most common congenital malformations of the head and neck.

1. **Cleft lip**

—with or without cleft palate occurs in 1 in 1000 newborns.

—may be associated with **poor feeding** and thus requires **early repair.**

—Classic criteria for timing of repair includes children 10 weeks of age and over 10 pounds.

2. **Cleft palate**

—generally does not require immediate repair.

—The timing of repair, however, depends on the risk of **poor speech de-velopment and swallowing without early repair** versus **abnor-mal maxillofacial growth with early repair.**

E. Branchial cleft cysts

—result from persistence of the embryologic branchial clefts.

1. The **second branchial cleft cyst** is the **most common** lesion.

    a. Second branchial clefts or fistulae

      —present as a mass **just anterior to the SCM** with a tract gener-ally passing between the internal and external carotids, ending in the tonsillar fossa.

    b. First branchial cleft lesions

      —may communicate with the external auditory canal.

      —are frequently closely associated with CN VII.

  2. Treatment

    —involves complete surgical excision.

F. Thyroglossal duct cysts

  —represent midline remnants of the embryologic descent of the thyroid from the base of the tongue.

  1. These present as a **midline cervical mass** and can contain normal thyroid tissue.

  2. Ultrasound or thyroid scanning

    —will help identify the location of the thyroid tissue in relation to the cyst.

  3. Treatment

    —involves **surgical resection** of the tract or cyst, which often requires resection of a portion of the hyoid bone.

VII. Trauma to the Head and Neck

A. Initial management

  —should always include the ABCs of trauma assessment (see *BRS General Surgery,* Chapter 8 I D).

B. Penetrating neck trauma (see BRS General Surgery, Chapter 8 V A)

C. Blunt neck trauma

  1. Laryngeal fracture

    a. This fracture is an airway emergency.

    b. Symptoms may include

      —ecchymosis.

      —**crepitus.**

      —stridor.

      —subcutaneous emphysema.

  2. Treatment

    a. No patient should be sedated until an airway has been secured.

    b. Subsequent surgical reconstruction is indicated.

D. Nerve injury

  1. Facial nerve injury may result from laceration, crush injury, or tem-poral bone fracture.

2. If a **temporal bone fracture occurs** the most common site of injury is at the **geniculate ganglion.**

3. **High-resolution CT scanning** of the region is useful in the evaluation.

4. **Temporal bone fractures** occur with significant impact to the skull.

   a. **Their orientation** to the **petrous ridge classifies** them as either **longitudinal** (80%) or **transverse** (20%).

   b. **Longitudinal fractures**

      —occur with lateral skull blows.

      —may be associated with **CN VII injury (20%)** or **conductive hearing loss** caused by ossicular chain disruption.

   c. **Transverse fractures**

      —occur with blows to the occiput.

      —are associated with **CN VII injury (50%)** and **sensorineural hearing loss** from CN VIII injury.

E. Soft tissue injuries

   —should be explored with aggressive irrigation and débridement of nonviable tissues.

F. Fractures

1. The **nasal bones** are the **most common** facial bones fractured.

   —Treatment is aimed at reduction of the fractured segments for cosmesis.

2. The **mandible**

   —is the **second** most commonly fractured facial bone. Symptoms are gross disfigurement, pain, malocclusion, and drooling.

   a. The **goal of treatment**

      —is to reestablish **normal occlusion.**

   b. **Occlusion is classified** as

      —**Class I:** normal.

      —**Class II:** overbite.

      —**Class III:** underbite.

   c. **Surgical treatment** involves either or both

      —maxillomandibular fixation (MMF).

      —open reduction internal fixation (ORIF) with plates or wires.

3. An **orbital blowout fracture**

   —occurs when a blow to the globe transmits energy to the weakest part of the orbit, the floor.

   a. **Treatment**

      —involves reconstruction of the floor only if there is significant diplopia and/or enophthalmos, causing cosmetic deformity.

   b. **Extraocular muscle entrapment**

      —is not considered a surgical emergency but needs to be evaluated.

4. **Midface fractures**

   a. The **Le Fort fractures** describe fractures of the midface **(Figure 4.5).**

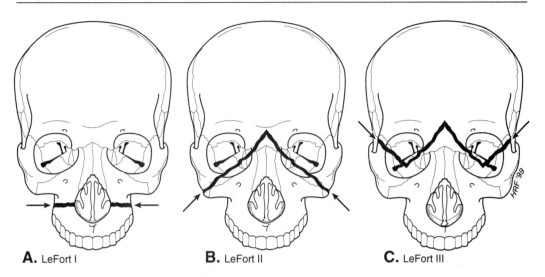

A. LeFort I   **B.** LeFort II   **C.** LeFort III

Figure 4.5. Le Fort fractures. (*A*) Le Fort type I is a transverse maxillary fracture. (*B*) Le Fort type II is a fracture through the maxilla, orbital floor, and pterygoid plate. (*C*) Le Fort type III (complete craniofacial separation) additionally extends through the nasofrontal and frontozygomatic sutures. (Adapted with permission from **Blackbourne** LH: *Surgical Recall.* Baltimore, Williams and Wilkins, 1994, pp 253–254.)

   b. Treatment involves
   —open reduction.
   —internal fixation for cosmesis.

5. **Tripod fractures**
   —are characterized by a complete fracture of the **zygomatic bone,** resulting in sunken cheeks.
   —**Treatment** involves open reduction and internal fixation for cosmesis.

Review Test

Directions: Each of the numbered items or incomplete statements in this section is followed by answers or by completions of the statement. Select the ONE lettered answer or completion that is BEST in each case.

1. A 34-year-old, previously healthy woman presents with a 2-week complaint of pressure and pain between her eyes and cheek, along with postnasal drip, nasal congestion, and anterior nasal greenish malodorous drainage. This is her first episode of these symptoms. She has no neurologic symptoms. Which of the following is the most appropriate next step in the diagnosis and management of this patient?

(A) Perform a sinus computed tomography (CT) scan
(B) Perform a cranial CT scan
(C) Maxillary sinus needle aspiration
(D) Nasal decongestant and antibiotics
(E) Observation alone

2. A 10-year-old boy presents to the office with a 4-month history of a right-sided draining ear and decreased hearing without significant pain. He has a past medical history of multiple episodes of otitis media (OM) as a child, which required pressure equalization (PE) tubes. The PE tubes fell out 5 years ago, and he has not had an ear infection since that time. He is afebrile. On physical examination his right ear canal is completely obstructed by mucopurulent material. The rest of his head and neck examination is normal. Which of the following is most appropriate in the diagnosis and management of this patient?

(A) Admit to hospital for intravenous (IV) antibiotics and treat for coalescent mastoiditis
(B) Suction the ear and remove the foreign body
(C) Place the patient on ear drops and treat for otitis externa
(D) Place the patient on oral antibiotics and treat for otitis media (OM)
(E) Clean the ear and examine for potential cholesteatoma

3. A 58-year-old man presents to the clinic with a 7-month history of a painless swelling behind the angle of the mandible on the left side. He is a nonsmoker and does not drink alcohol. He has never had this type of swelling before. He thinks that it may have grown slightly over the last few weeks but he cannot be sure. His head and neck examination is normal except for a 2-cm, firm, fixed mass in the location stated above. His neck is negative for adenopathy, and he denies any recent upper respiratory tract infection. Which of the following tissues most likely accounts for the mass noted in this patient?

(A) Salivary gland
(B) Skin
(C) Lymph node
(D) Mandible
(E) Ear cartilage

4. A 15-year-old young man presents to the clinic with a 2-month complaint of a hard mass in his mouth. The mass is nontender and does not bleed, there is no history of trauma, and the mass has not changed in size. He has no sinus complaints. Head and neck examination reveals a 1-cm hard smooth mucosal covered midline palate mass. There is no ulcer or erythema associated with the lesion. The rest of his oral cavity, oropharynx, and larynx are normal. His neck is negative for adenopathy. Which of the following would be the most appropriate next step in the management of this patient?

(A) Biopsy the lesion
(B) Take the patient to the operating room for surgical excision
(C) Perform a head computed tomography (CT) scan to rule out cranial tumor
(D) Work him up for gout
(E) Observation

5. A 32-year-old man presents to the emergency room with a 4-day complaint of right neck swelling, severe throat pain, fevers up to 103°F, stiff neck, pain with swallowing, and stridor. He also notes a 2-week history of a right tooth ache, although his symptoms have worsened in the last 24 hours. His head and neck examination reveals a large 6 × 7 cm, right-neck, firm swelling with overlaying skin induration. The patient is also noted to have trismus and can only open his mouth about 1 cm wide. He is unable to turn his neck because of pain, and his tongue appears normal. He is breathing with oxygen saturation above 97% on room air, but he has inspiratory and expiratory stridor. His chest radiograph is clear, and white blood cell count is 30,000. Which of the following would be the most appropriate next step in the management of this patient?

(A) Admit the patient and place him on intravenous (IV) antibiotics
(B) Culture his oral cavity and admit for IV antibiotics
(C) Administer IV morphine for pain control and obtain a computed tomography (CT) scan
(D) Perform nasotracheal intubation intraoperatively to secure the airway
(E) Perform a tracheostomy intraoperatively under local anesthesia

6. A 57-year-old woman presents to the clinic with a 6-month history of right ear pressure, high-pitched roaring, fluctuating hearing loss, and occasional dizzy spells. The dizzy spells are described as true vertigo, with the room spinning, that lasts about 45 minutes with associated nausea. She feels unsteady for a few hours after the episodes, and they occur about once every 2 weeks. She is a nonsmoker and nondrinker. She does not have a sinusitis history. She has a past medical history for depression and is on an antidepressant. The physical examination is negative for nystagmus, and ear examination is normal. An audiogram reveals a sensorineural, low-frequency, right-sided hearing loss. Which of the following would be the most appropriate next step in the management of this patient?

(A) Computed tomography (CT) scan to rule out brain tumor
(B) Low-salt diet and diuretic administration
(C) Discontinue the antidepressant medication
(D) Refer patient for neurologic work-up
(E) Perform a vertebral artery arteriogram

7. A 40-year-old woman presents to the clinic 1 week after an uncomplicated, right-sided, superficial parotidectomy for a presumed pleomorphic adenoma. The final pathology report gives the diagnosis of a high-grade mucoepidermoid carcinoma with a 1-mm close margin. Which of the following is the most appropriate advice for this patient?

(A) The tumor was completely removed and no more treatment is required
(B) A total parotidectomy alone is adequate
(C) Postoperative adjuvant radiation therapy alone is adequate
(D) A total parotidectomy with postoperative chemotherapy is adequate
(E) A total parotidectomy with postoperative radiation therapy is adequate

Answers and Explantations

1-D. The scenario described suggests an episode of acute sinusitis. Antibiotics and nasal decongestants are the most appropriate treatment for an initial episode of infection. Sinus computed tomography (CT) scan is reserved for patients with recurrent acute sinusitis (multiple episodes of acute sinusitis with asymptomatic periods) or chronic sinusitis (symptoms lasting longer than 4 weeks). There is no indication for a head CT unless neurologic symptoms are present. Needle aspiration of the sinus is usually reserved for chronic sinusitis. Observation alone is inadequate because of the potential risk of complications including orbital abscess, meningitis, brain abscess, and sigmoid sinus thrombosis.

2-E. The patient's history and physical examination are most consistent with a possible right-sided cholesteatoma. The initial treatment consists of cleaning the ear to identify the tympanic membrane and location of possible cholesteatoma perforating the tympanic membrane. This is followed by an audiogram to document hearing, and then treating the child with antibiotic ear drops and dry ear precautions to clear the ear of drainage. A middle ear exploration with removal of the cholesteatoma in the operating room is the definitive treatment. A foreign body is generally associated with significant pain, as is otitis externa. An otitis media (OM) is also frequently associated with pain as well as fever. Coalescent mastoiditis is generally associated with fever, with pain, fluctuance, and erythema noted over the mastoid.

3-A. The history and physical examination is most consistent with a tumor of the tail of the parotid gland. The patient's age, gender, and essentially asymptomatic presentation would be most consistent with pleomorphic adenoma or Warthin's tumor of the parotid. A sebaceous cyst of the skin is possible but should have presented at a younger age with intermittent swelling and infections. A high anterior cervical lymphadenopathy could develop after an upper respiratory tract infection, which the patient did not have. A metastatic node is unlikely with a negative smoking and drinking history, and a good head and neck examination should localize the lesion to the parotid. A mandible lesion would generally be fixed to the mandible. Lesions of the ear are uncommon and would not be found in the location described.

4-E. The patient's history and physical examination are most consistent with a torus palatinus. This is a midline hard palate bony mass that is a normal variant. Torus mandibulare are similar lesions located on the anterior inner table of the mandible, and are frequently bilateral. A biopsy is not indicated for these lesions, nor is surgical excision. It is likely this has been present for many years but the patient was not aware or did not pay attention to the mass. There are a number of midline head and neck lesions, but they are associated with other symptoms such as pain, friability, and bleeding. These lesions are not associated with gout or intracranial tumors.

5-E. This patient's history and physical examination is most consistent with a deep neck abscess of dental origin. Stridor is a sign of possible airway compromise, and airway stabilization is the first consideration. A patient with trismus cannot be orally intubated, so nasotracheal intubation is possible but visualization of the pharynx would be difficult. The correct answer is local tracheostomy to secure the airway, followed by external neck drainage of the abscess. Culture of the oral cavity would be of no benefit. Never administer pain medications or sedatives to a patient with potential airway compromise because this could reduce the patient's respiratory drive and lead to complete airway obstruction.

6-B. The patient's history is classic for Ménière's disease. Unilateral aural fullness, tinnitus, fluctuating low-frequency hearing loss, and spells of vertigo lasting more than 20 minutes are diagnostic for this disease. A computed tomography (CT) scan would only be indicated if the patient had other neurologic symptoms. Depression can cause dizziness, lightheadedness, and vertigo, along with many other symptoms, but Ménière's disease is the most likely diagnosis, given her history. A neurologic referral is not indicated. The first line of treatment for Ménière's disease is a low-salt diet, diuretic administration, and a vestibular suppressant such as meclizine. A vertebral artery arteriogram is not indicated in the work-up of this patient.

7-E. The treatment of intermediate and high-grade mucoepidermoid carcinomas of the salivary glands is total parotidectomy with postoperative adjuvant radiation therapy. A neck dissection may also be indicated, depending on physician preference. These tumors are considered aggressive and a 1-mm margin is too close, therefore adjuvant therapy is indicated. Chemotherapy plays little or no role in the treatment of these tumors.

5

Orthopedics

Abhinav Chhabra, Todd A. Milbrandt

I. Trauma

A. Definitions

1. Fracture descriptions

a. Fractures may be classified

—based on the anatomic location and the type of fracture as outlined in **Figure 5.1.**

b. Segmental fractures

—are characterized by a large interspersed fragment.

c. Characterization of the fracture site deformity

—is also outlined in **Figure 5.1.**

(1) The **direction** of **fracture displacement** is defined by the relative relationship of the **distal** fragment to the proximal fragment (i.e., posterior, anterior, medial, and lateral).

(2) The **degree of displacement** is measured in relation to the thickness of the shaft (i.e., displaced half the diameter of the shaft medially).

(3) **Pathologic fractures** occur at sites of **infection or tumor,** usually resulting from a low energy injury because of poor bone quality.

(4) A **stress fracture** results from weakness of bone secondary to repetitive low energy trauma.

(5) A **greenstick fracture** is an incomplete fracture of one cortex only, commonly seen in children.

2. Other definitions

a. Torus: buckling of the metaphyseal cortex seen in children (i.e., distal radius)

b. Nonunion: no callus or radiologic healing of the fracture within 9 months after injury

123

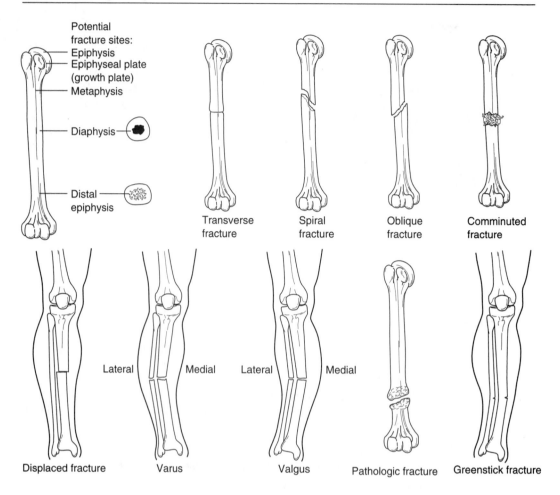

Figure 5.1. Fracture descriptions. (Adapted with permission from Blackbourne LH: *Surgical Recall.* Baltimore, Williams & Wilkins, 1994, pp 299–306.)

    c. Delayed union: minimal callus formation and healing 3–9 months after injury

    d. Malunion: healing of fracture in an angulated or rotated position

    e. Reduction: re-alignment of the segments in a fracture via closed manipulation or by surgical means (correction of the deformity)

    f. Dislocation: disruption of a joint, often associated with ligamentous and bony injury

B. Evaluation of fractures

    1. During the secondary survey

        a. After evaluation of the ABCs

            —(see *BRS General Surgery*, Chapter 8 I D 1), the extremities can be addressed.

        b. The key signs of a fracture are

            —pain.

            —swelling.

—deformity.

—crepitus.

—instability.

2. Anterior-posterior and lateral radiographs

—of the involved extremity should be performed.

C. Open fractures

1. An open fracture has a **direct communication with the external environment through the skin.**

—This increases the risk of osteomyelitis and poor fracture healing.

2. A classification system for open fractures is outlined in **Table 5-1.**

3. Treatment

—is focused on infection prevention and bony realignment.

a. Initial and repeated **irrigation and débridement** of devitalized tissues

b. Broad spectrum antibiotics and tetanus immunization particularly for dirty or soiled wounds

c. Fracture stabilization

d. Delayed primary wound closure or **skin and muscle flap** coverage for large soft tissue defects

D. Associated vascular injury

1. Vascular injury must be suspected

—with any major fracture or fracture-dislocation.

2. Classic findings in the injury include

—pallor.

—pulselessness.

—paralysis.

—cool temperature.

3. Evaluation should include

Table 5-1. Gustilo and Anderson Classification of Open Fractures

Grade	Description
I	<1 cm soft tissue laceration
II	>1 cm, but <10 cm soft tissue laceration with moderate contamination
IIIA	>10 cm soft tissue defect with high contamination
IIIB	>10 cm soft tissue defect with periosteal stripping and high contamination
IIIC	Grade III A or B with vascular compromise

—blood pressure monitoring with calculation of the ankle-brachial index (see Chapter 1 III A 1).

—**doppler** examination of the pulses in the affected extremity.

—an **arteriogram,** when the diagnosis is uncertain or when anatomic localization is needed.

4. **Treatment**

—involves **immediate reduction of the fracture** or dislocation followed by **reassessment for the return of perfusion.**

a. Once **reperfusion has been established,** stabilization of the fracture is required.

b. With **severe arterial injuries, vascular repair or bypass grafting** may be needed.

E. **Traumatic long bone fractures**

—may result in **fat emboli syndrome** (see *BRS General Surgery,* Chapter 2 III H 5), which results in acute respiratory distress syndrome (ARDS).

F. **Compartment syndrome**

—may also develop following extremity fractures (see *BRS General Surgery,* Chapter 5 III F).

1. **Clinical presentation**

a. The **classic finding** is **pain with passive stretch of the involved muscle compartment.**

b. **Other findings** include

—pallor.

—pulselessness.

—paresthesia.

—paralysis.

2. **Compartment syndrome most commonly develops after**

—supracondylar humeral fractures.

—tibial fractures.

—crush injuries.

3. **Diagnosis is based on the history and physical examination findings.**

—**Compartment** pressures may be measured to confirm the diagnosis, with values over 30–40 mm Hg considered elevated (normal < 20 mm Hg).

4. **Treatment**

a. In the affected area, decompression of all fascia-contained muscular compartments via fasciotomy is required.

b. **Complications of delayed diagnosis** (longer than 6–8 hours) include ischemic contractures and severe neurovascular injury.

c. **Volkmann's contractures** result from ischemia of the flexor muscles of the forearm, most commonly after a supracondylar humeral fracture.

G. Treatment of fractures

1. Initial splinting

—is necessary for pain relief and stabilization during transport.

2. Closed versus open reduction

a. Closed reduction

—involves external manipulation of the extremity to realign the fractured segments.

—After reduction, a cast or splint is applied to provide immobilization.

b. Open reduction

—involves **surgical manipulation** and stabilization of displaced fracture segments.

(1) Operative fixation may be accomplished with intramedullary nails or plate and screw fixation **(Figures 5.2 and 5.3).**

(2) Fractures that involve the articular surface of any joint are best treated with open reduction and anatomic realignment of the joint line.

3. External fixation (Figure 5.4)

a. Uses **pins** through the skin that are attached to external bars or rings to stabilize the reduced fracture

b. Indications

—Open fractures with extensive bone and soft tissue loss associated with an increased infection risk

4. Traction

a. Traction immobilization

—uses weights to overcome the distracting force of the muscles around the fracture to maintain correct alignment.

b. Skeletal traction

—may be applied to the lower extremity through a femoral, tibial, or calcaneal pin, thereby temporarily stabilizing the fracture.

c. Definitive treatment with skeletal traction

—is limited to **femur fractures in infants and children.**

H. Characteristics of specific fractures and dislocations

—are listed in **Tables 5-2 and 5-3**

II. Sports-Related Injuries

A. Rotator cuff injury

1. The **rotator cuff consists** of **four muscles of the shoulder** (SITS acronym)

—supraspinatus.

—infraspinatus.

—teres minor.

—subscapularis.

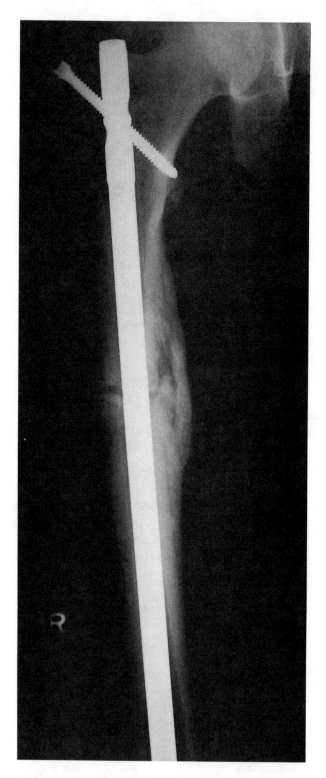

Figure 5.2. Fixation of femoral shaft fracture with intramedullary nailing.

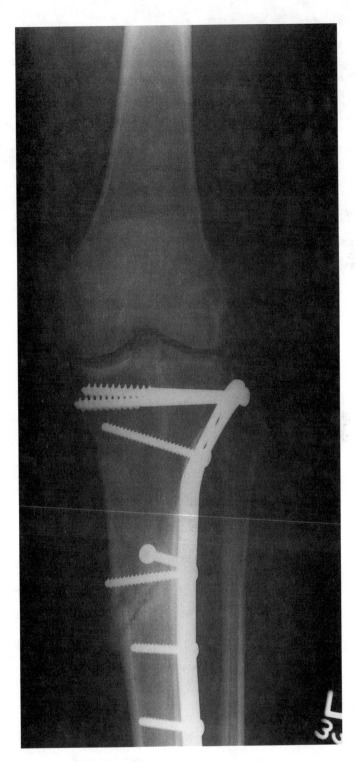

Figure 5.3. Plate and screw fixation of a proximal fracture of the tibia.

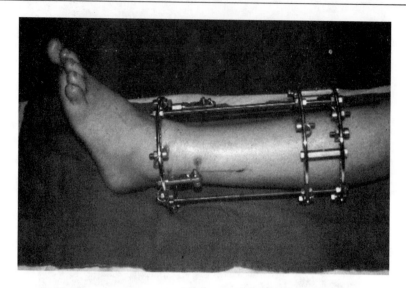

Figure 5.4. Fixation of tibia fracture with external fixation.

Table 5-2. Upper Extremity Fractures and Dislocations

Fracture/ Dislocation	Radiologic Evaluation	Treatment	Complications
Clavicle	AP view of the clavicle; most occur in the mid to distal ⅓	Figure of 8 brace; surgery only for skin compromise, vascular impingement, or nonunion	Cosmetic deformity or nonunion
Acromioclavicular joint dislocation	AP view of the acromioclavicular joint	Sling and swath; surgery for severe displacement	Brachial plexus and vascular injury
Scapula	AP and scapular-Y view	Sling and immobilization; internal fixation if glenoid involved	Associated with thoracic aortic injury, hemo-pneumothorax
Shoulder dislocation	AP, lateral, and axillary views (anterior: 90%) (posterior: 10%)	Closed reduction followed by repeat films to evaluate for fracture, followed by 3 weeks in sling; surgery if unable to reduce or if displaced fracture of proximal humerus	Axillary nerve and brachial plexus damage, fracture of the proximal humerus, recurrent dislocations; posterior dislocation seen with seizures
Proximal humerus/ shaft	AP, lateral, and axillary views	Sling for nondisplaced fractures; surgery for displaced, comminuted fractures	Axillary nerve damage

(*continued*)

Table 5-2. Upper Extremity Fractures and Dislocations

Fracture/ Dislocation	Radiologic Evaluation	Treatment	Complications
Humeral shaft	AP and lateral views	Coaptation splint followed by a fracture brace at 2 weeks; surgery for failed reduction or neurovascular deficits	Axillary nerve damage; oblique/spiral distal ⅓ shaft fractures **(Holstein/Lewis)** have increased risk of radial nerve injury
Supracondylar humerus	AP and lateral views	In children, closed reduction and casting unless largely displaced or comminuted; surgery via Kirshner wires; adults treated with internal fixation	Brachial artery and median/radial nerve at increased risk of **Volkmann's contracture**
Elbow dislocation and fracture	AP and lateral views	Immediate reduction if dislocated followed by cast placement or surgery if comminuted; early motion is key	Ulnar and radial nerve damage
Forearm fracture	AP and lateral views	In adults, if both the radius and the ulna are broken, operative treatment is required; in children, closed reduction and casting is preferred	Ulnar and radial nerve damage
Distal radius (most common fracture in children)	AP and lateral views **Colles:** dorsally displaced **Smith:** volarly displaced	Reduction is attempted followed by splint placement; surgery for failed reductions, articular incongruity, or neurovascular involvement	Acute carpal tunnel syndrome; post-traumatic arthritis
Wrist (scaphoid, lunate)	AP, lateral, and scaphoid views	Pain in the anatomic snuffbox is key for scaphoid fracture; most are treated in cast immobilization; displaced scaphoid fractures and lunate dislocations require internal fixation	If lunate is dislocated, then there is a high risk for **Keinbock's disease,** avascular necrosis of the lunate

AP = anterior–posterior (view).

2. Rotator cuff tear may result from

—an acute traumatic event or a chronic degeneration of the tendons.

  a. This often **presents** with shoulder pain and decreased range of motion.

Table 5-3. Lower Extremity Fractures or Dislocations

Fracture/ Dislocation	Radiologic Evaluation	Treatment	Complications
Pelvic fractures	AP, lateral, inlet, and outlet views; and CT scan	Pelvic hemorrhage controlled with external fixation and angiographic embolization; pelvic reconstruction performed when hemodynamically stable; single rami fractures treated with gradual weight bearing	Life-threatening hemorrhage, urogenital disruption; frequently associated with other severe injuries (e.g., intra-abdominal)
Hip dislocations	AP and lateral films; posterior dislocation most common	Immediate reduction under conscious sedation	Sciatic nerve damage, acetabular fractures, and femoral neck fractures (10% risk of avascular necrosis of the femoral head)
Femoral neck	AP and lateral films; MRI for occult fractures	Internal fixation or hemiarthroplasty (partial joint replacement)	Avascular necrosis risk high with large displacement
Femoral shaft	AP and lateral films	Children: cast application Adults: intramedullary nailing	Malunion and nonunion
Patella	AP and lateral films	Nondisplaced fractures: long-leg cast Comminuted fractures: internal fixation	Avascular necrosis of the patella, loss of extension of the knee
Tibial shaft	AP and lateral films	Most treated with intramedullary rod; open fractures: external fixation	Compartment syndrome, nonunion, malunion
Ankle injuries	AP, lateral, and 30-degree mortise views	Ligamentous injuries: rest and pain control Stable fractures: cast immobilization Bi- or trimalleolar fractures: ORIF	Post-traumatic arthritis
Talus	AP and lateral films	Reduction with cast placement for most; severe displacement: internal fixation; early motion helps prevent a stiff ankle	Avascular necrosis is common
Calcaneus	AP and lateral films, and CT scan	Nondisplaced fractures: nonweight-bearing and casting; all others require internal fixation	Compartment syndrome of the foot; 10% associated with lumbar spine fractures

(continued)

Table 5-3. Lower Extremity Fractures or Dislocations

Fracture/ Dislocation	Radiologic Evaluation	Treatment	Complications
Metatarsal	AP and lateral films of the foot; watch for **Jones fracture** (fracture of the fifth metatarsal)	Decrease activity level with cast immobiliz-ation or fracture brace for 4–6 weeks; surgery with failed conserva-tive management	Nonunion is common after a Jones fracture, requiring internal fixation

AP = anterior–posterior (view); CT = computed tomography; MRI = magnetic resonance imaging (scan); ORIF = open reduction and internal fixation.

b. These occur most often in the fifth decade.

3. **Physical examination** often reveals

—**weakness to internal and external rotation.**

—**abduction of the arm.**

4. **Evaluation**

—Radiographs of the shoulder should be used to rule out fracture.

—**Magnetic resonance imaging (MRI)** is used to characterize the extent of muscular and soft tissue injury.

5. **Treatment**

a. For **acute tears**

—**Placement of a sling** is initially appropriate until the pain resolves.

—Surgical repair should be attempted when the patient needs to return to a high level of activity (i.e., pitching) or in active individuals in which the activities of daily living are compromised.

b. **Chronic tears**

—can be treated conservatively with physical therapy for muscle strengthening and early range-of-motion exercises.

B. **Ligamentous injuries to the knee**

1. **Medial and lateral collateral ligaments (MCL and LCL)**

a. **Injuries** to the

—**MCL** occur after **valgus stress,** or pressure on the lateral portion of the knee (see Figure 5.1).

—**LCL** occur after **varus stress,** or pressure on the medial portion of the knee.

b. **MCL and LCL injuries** are often associated with meniscus or cruciate ligament injuries.

c. **Patients generally present** with knee pain and difficulty ambulating.

d. **Findings**

—For **MCL injuries,** valgus stress causes medial opening of the knee joint.

—For **LCL injuries,** varus stress will show lateral opening of the knee joint.

e. **Diagnosis**

—**Plain films** should be taken to rule out fractures.

—**MRI** will demonstrate the injured soft tissues.

f. **Treatment** depends on the size of the injury.

—**Small MCL tears** are often treated in a brace.

—**Large MCL tears require surgical repair.**

—LCL tears often require surgical repair.

2. **Anterior cruciate ligament (ACL) injury**

a. **Injury to the ACL occurs with pivoting** actions.

b. **Women athletes** are at increased risk for ACL injuries.

c. **Patients often present** with **knee pain and a joint effusion.**

d. **Diagnosis**

(1) A positive **anterior drawer test**

—is elicited by **forward displacement of the tibia** with respect to the femur with the knee flexed to 90°.

—Comparison to the uninjured knee is essential.

(2) **Lachman's test**

—is more specific for ACL injuries.

—is characterized by forward displacement of the tibia with the knee flexed to 30°.

(3) **Plain films**

—**should be performed** to rule out fracture.

e. **When the diagnosis is in question,** an **MRI** may be performed.

—Associated meniscal and other ligamentous injuries may be identified.

f. **Treatment**

(1) In an **active person with instability of the knee**

—**surgical reconstruction** with a portion of patella tendon or hamstring tendon graft is indicated.

(2) An **inactive patient**

—may be treated with physical therapy for muscle strengthening and bracing.

3. **Posterior cruciate ligament (PCL) injury**

a. **PCL injury is rare,** although it may be associated with knee dislocation.

b. **Patients often present** with knee pain and a joint effusion.

c. **Injuries to the ACL and the LCL** are characteristically associated with PCL injuries.

d. **Diagnosis**

(1) The **posterior drawer test** associated with PCL injury demonstrates **posterior displacement of the tibia** with respect to the femur with the knee flexed 90°.

(2) Plain films help to rule out fracture.

(3) MRI is generally diagnostic.

e. Treatment

(1) Patients may be treated conservatively with **physical therapy for muscle strengthening and bracing.**

(2) Surgical reconstruction is indicated in active patients who fail conservative management.

4. Meniscal injuries

a. These injuries **generally result from traumatic twisting of the knee.** They may also result from degenerative changes seen in osteoarthritis.

b. A **"locking" or "catching" sensation** is pathognomonic for a meniscal tear.

c. Diagnosis

(1) On **physical examination**

—medial or lateral joint line tenderness is often present.

(2) The **McMurray test**

—is classically used for meniscal evaluation.

(a) For this test the knee is flexed and the foot is placed in internal or external rotation.

(b) The knee is then gradually extended, feeling for a **click or pop, or pain along the medial or lateral joint line.**

(3) Plain films

—help to rule out fracture.

(4) MRI

—can help discern occult meniscal injuries.

d. Treatment

(1) The **outer rim is the only vascular portion of the meniscus.**

—If a **tear occurs in** or **through the rim,** arthroscopic repair is indicated.

(2) In **tears not amenable to repair,** arthroscopic débridement will often relieve the symptoms.

III. Pediatric Orthopedics

A. Growth plate injury

1. Description

a. These injuries are usually the **result** of trauma or infection.

b. They are **classified** according to the

—involvement of the physis, metaphysis, and epiphysis.

—degree of displacement.

—See **Figure 5.5.** for the Salter-Harris classification.

2. Radiographic evaluation

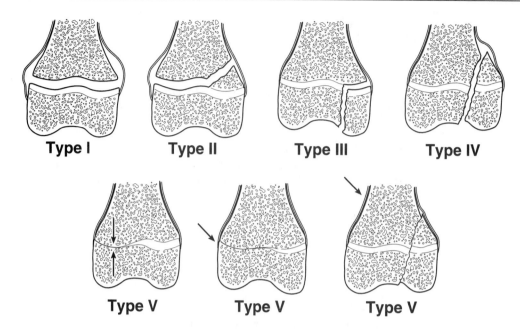

Figure 5.5. Salter-Harris classification of growth plate injuries. *Type I:* fracture through the growth plate. *Type II:* fracture along the growth plate and metaphysis. *Type III:* fracture along the growth plate and epiphysis. *Type IV:* fracture along the growth plate and through the epiphysis and metaphysis. *Type V:* crush injury to the growth plate. (Adapted with permission from Morrissy R (ed): *Lowell and Winter's Pediatric Orthopaedics.* Philadelphia, Lippincott, 1990, p 777.)

    a. Anterior-posterior (AP) and lateral radiographs of the involved extremity are generally diagnostic.

    b. Radiographs performed while applying stress to the extremity may also be useful.

  3. Treatment

    a. The **goal of treatment**

      —is to return the growth plate to its anatomic position.

    b. Severe injury

      —can result in **leg length discrepancy** or angular deformity.

    c. Salter-Harris I/II injuries

      —can be treated with **closed reduction and casting.**

    d. Salter-Harris III/IV injuries

      —require **open reduction or internal fixation.**

    e. Treatment

      —**should be followed** for 2 years after injury to ensure that neither an angular deformity nor leg length discrepancy develops.

B. Osteomyelitis

  1. This **infection is commonly seen** in children in the metaphysis of long bones.

    —Most common organism is a staphylococcal species.

  2. Children present with pain and decreased use of the involved extremity.

3. **Evaluation**

—Serum erythrocyte sedimentation rate

—Blood cultures

—AP and lateral films

—MRI

—**Bone biopsy** for identification of the causative organism.

4. **Treatment**

—**Irrigation and débridement** of devitalized bone in addition to administration of intravenous (IV) antibiotics are included in the treatment.

C. **Cerebral palsy** (CP)

—affects 1/1000 children.

1. **Factors that have been implicated** include

—head injury.

—anoxic events.

—encephalitis.

—prenatal viral illnesses.

2. **Definitions**
   a. **Diplegic:** motor abnormality of lower extremities
   b. **Hemiplegic:** motor abnormality involving one side of the body
   c. **Quadriplegic:** motor abnormality of all four limbs
   d. **Athetosis:** dyskinesia characterized by purposeless writhing movements
   e. **Ataxic:** disturbance of coordinated movement most notable when walking
   f. **Spastic:** diffuse increase in muscle tone

3. Among patients with CP, the **distribution** of the different types include

—50% **spastic form.**

—25% **athetoid form.**

—5% **ataxic form.**

—The remainder are a mixed type.

4. **Paralysis accompanies the spasticity in most cases.**

5. CP patients may suffer from **multiple problems** including

—scoliosis.

—hip subluxation.

—soft tissue contractures.

6. **Treatment**
   a. In the absence of a cure for CP, the **cornerstones of treatment** are
      —muscle strengthening.
      —physiotherapy.

—gait training.

—proper orthotic use.

b. Surgical intervention

(1) Surgery may be considered for progressive scoliosis or for severe contracture resulting in significant alteration of daily activities.

(2) Surgical procedures include

—adductor release.

—hamstring/Achilles tendon lengthening for severe contractures.

—spinal fusion for progressive scoliosis.

—femoral/acetabular osteotomies for hip subluxation.

D. Idiopathic adolescent scoliosis (Figure 5.6)

1. Scoliosis

—represents an **abnormal curvature of the spine.**

—occurs **most frequently in prepubertal females.**

2. The **most common type of idiopathic scoliosis** is a **right thoracic curve.**

—The **primary curve** is defined by the longest curve with the greatest degree of angulation.

3. Most patients are asymptomatic, although **backache or fatigue** may rarely be present.

—Physical examination may show rib hump while the patient is flexed at the waist.

4. Radiologic evaluation

—Standing AP, lateral, and lateral bending films are required to evaluate the curve thoroughly.

5. Treatment

a. In **prepubertal patients**

—**curves between 20°–45° require bracing** to slow progression.

—Progression of disease may occur during the pubertal growth spurt.

b. Curves greater than 45°

—or those with high likelihood of progression require **spinal fusion** with instrumentation and bone grafting.

E. Osgood-Schlatter disease

—is also called tibial tubercle apophysitis, or "growing pains."

1. This disease

—is caused by traction injury from the quadriceps muscle.

—generally affects **adolescents 13–15 years old.**

2. The **most common complaint**

—is **pain over the front of the knee.**

3. Examination

—Patients will frequently have pain over the tibial tubercle associated with direct palpation or with extension of the knee.

4. Radiographs

—may show an irregular or fragmented tibial tubercle.

5. Treatment

—**Mild symptoms:** simple restriction from aggressive activity

—**Severe symptoms:** cast application for 6 weeks, followed by activity modification

F. Legg-Calvé-Perthes disease (avascular necrosis of femoral head) [Figure 5.7]

1. This **disease results from** idiopathic **vascular insult** to the femoral head.

   —The vascular insult may be secondary to an underlying hypercoagulable state (e.g., protein C or S deficiency).

2. This **disease affects** children 2 years of age and older.

   —It is bilateral in **10%** of patients.

3. **Patients generally present** with **painful gait and limp.**

4. Radiologic evaluation

   —AP and lateral films of both hips will show progressive flattening of the femoral head with fragmentation.

5. **Treatment**

   a. The **cornerstone of treatment** for this disorder is to maintain range-of-motion and coverage of the femoral head.

   b. **Conservative treatment**

      —Limited weight bearing, physical therapy, and range-of-motion exercises are used.

      —Usually the femoral head remodels over time with no residual sequelae.

   c. **Surgical intervention**

      —To maintain coverage of the femoral head in the acetabulum, osteotomies or soft tissue release may be required if the conservative measures have failed or if the disease is too advanced.

G. Slipped capital femoral epiphysis (SCFE) [Figure 5.8]

1. This **disease generally affects** males **12–15 years** of age and females **10–13 years** of age.

   —It is **five times more common in males** and is more common in African-Americans.

2. There is an **increased risk for avascular necrosis of the femoral head.**

3. **Physical examination**

   —reveals an **antalgic (painful) gait** and pain with range of motion at the hip.

4. **Radiologic evaluation**

   —with an AP pelvis and bilateral lateral hip films will show widening and irregularity of the epiphyseal plate.

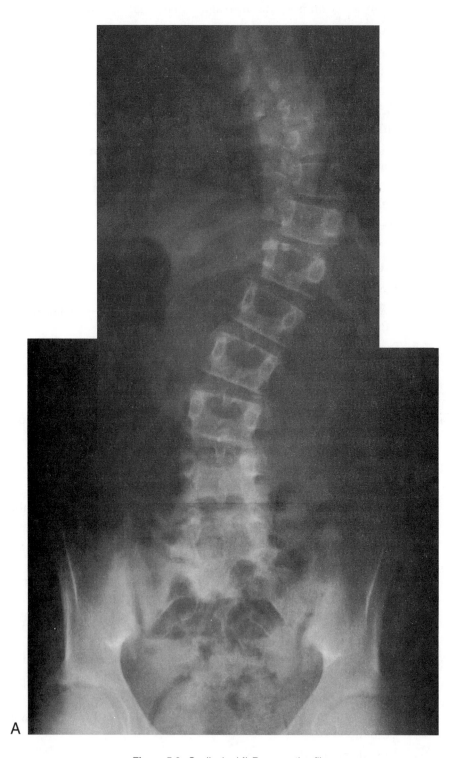

Figure 5.6. Scoliosis. (*A*) Preoperative film.

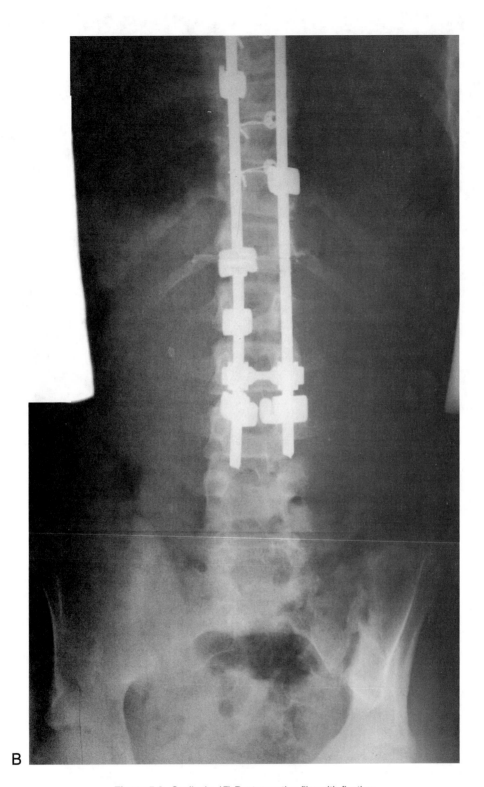

Figure 5.6. Scoliosis. (*B*) Postoperative film with fixation.

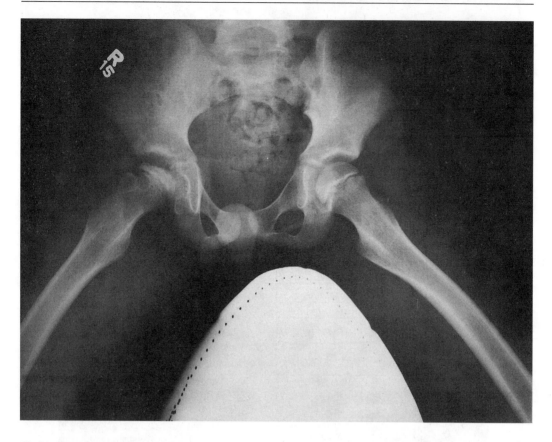

Figure 5.7. Legg-Calvé-Perthes disease as shown on anterior-posterior radiograph. Note the flattening of the femoral head on the right.

—The lateral views will show posterior subluxation of the epiphysis.

5. Treatment

—involves surgical pinning of the epiphysis in situ to prevent further slippage.

H. Congenital dislocations of the hip

1. This **occurs more commonly** in **female, first-born, and breech presentation babies.**

2. **Most dislocations are found** during post-natal exam and are bilateral **10% of the time.**

3. **Undiagnosed dislocations** that progress to an older age typically present with

   —pain.

   —abnormal gait.

   —early degenerative arthrosis.

4. Evaluation

   a. Subluxation of the hip

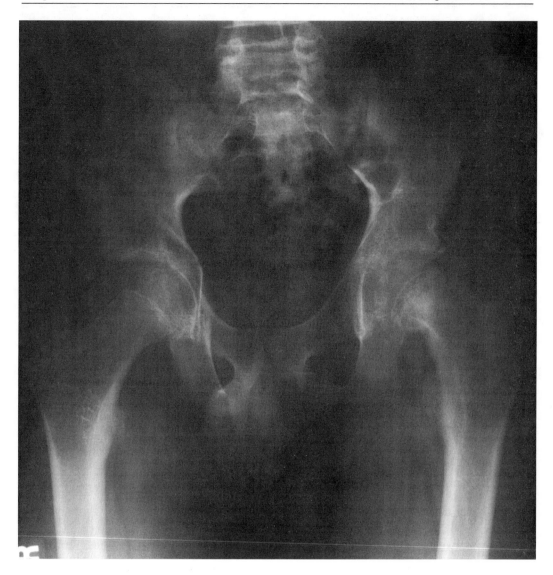

Figure 5.8. Slipped capital femoral epiphysis as seen on anterior-posterior radiograph of the pelvis. Note the asymmetry between the right and left femoral heads. The left femoral epiphysis has "slipped" from its normal anatomic position.

    —**when flexed to 90°** with direct pressure dorsally is considered a positive **Barlow's test.** Examiner can feel a "click".

b. Reduction of the subluxation

    —with direct pressure and abduction of the hip is considered a positive **Ortolani's test.**

c. Plain films

    —are difficult to interpret in an infant because the femoral head is not ossified.

d. Ultrasound

    —may be used to confirm the dislocation in neonates.

5. **Treatment**
   a. If the **dislocation is recognized early,** placement of a **Pavlik harness for 3–6 months** is usually adequate treatment.
      —The Pavlik harness keeps the legs flexed and abducted and the femoral head reduced in the acetabulum.
   b. **Placing a cast**
      —may also play a role if the harness does not correct the tendency to dislocate.
   c. **Operative treatment**
      —with surgical reduction of the hip and acetabular or femoral osteotomy is rarely indicated before 1 year of age.

I. **Clubfoot** (talipes equinovalgus)
   1. **Clubfoot is characterized** by
      —plantar flexion of the ankle.
      —supination of the foot.
      —adduction of the forefoot.
      —medial rotation of the tibia.
   2. **Plain radiographs**
      —are useful for evaluating the degree of malformation.
   3. The most effective **treatment** involves serial casting of the leg and foot at birth.
   4. **Surgical correction** consisting of muscle transfer and tenotomy may be performed at 6 months.

IV. Joint Diseases

A. **Septic (pyogenic) arthritis**
   1. **Joints may become infected** from many routes including
      —hematogenous spread.
      —direct infection.
      —extension from adjacent osteomyelitis.
   2. **Diagnosis**
      a. **Aspiration of the joint**
         —should be performed for culture and Gram stain.
      b. **Blood work**
         —should include white blood cell count and sedimentation rate.
      c. **Plain films, an MRI, or both**
         —may be useful for demonstrating joint destruction.
   3. A **septic joint** is a **surgical emergency**
      —requiring operative drainage of the involved joint followed by IV antibiotics.

B. Bony tuberculosis

1. This is a **very uncommon infection** in the United States, although there has recently been an increase in cases.

2. **Tuberculosis of the spine** and the extremities is **always secondary to a pulmonary infection.**

3. The **most common site** of skeletal infection is the **spine (Pott's disease).**

4. **Evaluation**

   —Erythrocyte sedimentation rate

   —Blood cultures

   —Bone biopsy looking for acid-fast bacilli

   —In addition, radiographs of the involved bone should be taken.

5. **Treatment**

   —involves surgical debridement and multi-drug therapy against tuberculosis.

C. Rheumatoid arthritis (RA)

—may affect any joint.

—is considered a systemic disease.

1. This **disease is more common** in **women (3:1)** and peaks between ages **30–40.**

2. Although the **etiology of RA is unknown,** pathologic features include congested and edematous tendons, bursa, and **synovium.**

   —Within the joint, the synovium invades the subchondral bone and initiates joint destruction.

3. **Patients typically present** with **stiffness** of the hands or affected joints **in the morning** or **after periods of inactivity.**

4. **Evaluation**
   a. **Serum rheumatoid factor**
      —is frequently elevated.
   b. **Physical examination**
      —may reveal subcuticular nodules and deformities of the fingers.
   c. **Plain films**
      —will show joint destruction and subluxation.

5. **Treatment**
   a. **Medical therapy** includes
      —**nonsteroidal anti-inflammatory drugs (NSAIDs).**
      —**steroids.**
      —**methotrexate.**
   b. **Operative treatment**
      —including **synovectomy or joint fusion or joint replacement may be performed if conservative measures fail** to alleviate pain.

   c. Figure 5-9 demonstrates a postoperative radiograph following a total knee replacement.

D. Gout

—is a metabolic disease where crystals of **sodium urate monohydrate** are deposited in joints.

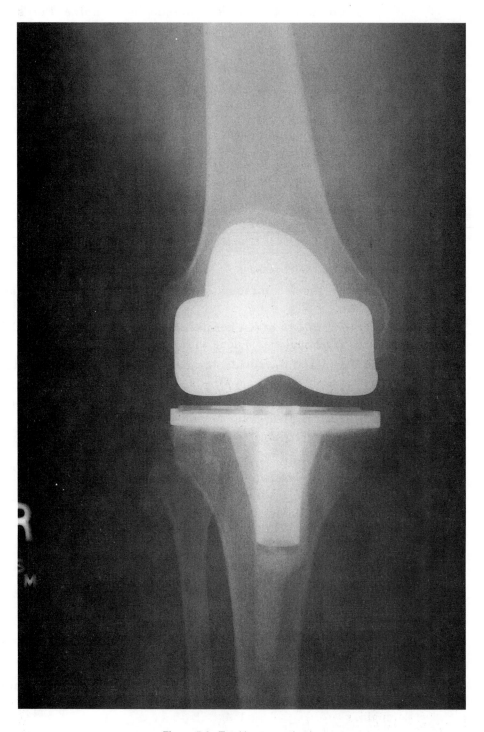

Figure 5.9. Total knee prosthesis.

—is commonly associated with **alcohol abuse.**

1. Primary and secondary gout

   a. Primary gout

     —is due to an **inborn error in metabolism of purine.**

   b. Secondary gout

     —is associated with other disease states such as **leukemia, hemolytic anemia, or myeloproliferative disease.**

2. The **most common site** of involvement is the **first metatarsal joint.**

3. Diagnosis

   a. Joint aspiration

     —will reveal crystals that are **negatively birefringent in polarized light.**

   b. Radiographs

     —may demonstrate soft tissue inflammation and joint destruction.

4. Treatment

   a. Acute attacks

     —Colchicine and indomethacin may be administered.

   b. Chronic disease

     —Allopurinol may be used.

E. Degenerative joint disease (osteoarthritis)

—is a slowly progressive disorder of one or many joints seen in normal aging.

1. This **disease principally affects load-bearing joints** (i.e., hip, knee, shoulder).

2. Although the **etiology is unknown,** the disease is associated with significant cartilage loss and destruction.

3. Characteristic findings include

—pain.

—swelling.

—joint deformity.

—limitation of the range of motion of the joint.

4. Radiographs may reveal

—loss of joint space.

—subchondral cysts.

—osteophytes.

5. Treatment

   a. Conservative measures for **osteoarthritis include**

     —NSAIDs.

     —steroid intra-articular injection.

     —physical therapy.

     —activity modification.

   b. Failure of conservative measures

     —is an indication for **total joint replacement.**

V. Generalized Bone Disorders

A. Achondroplasia

—is an **autosomal dominant disorder of the growth plate.**

1. At birth these children have a normal sized body but short and fat limbs.
2. The trunk remains unaffected.

B. Osteogenesis imperfecta

1. Osteogenesis imperfecta is **a defect in type I collagen** inherited as an autosomal dominant trait.
2. This disease is characterized by an extreme **fragility of bones** and an increased tendency to fracture.

C. Osteopetrosis

—is a defect in osteoclast function inherited as an autosomal **recessive trait.**

1. This **disease** is **characterized by** an increased density of the skeleton because of increased calcification of osteoid tissues.

   —The **bone,** however, **is very brittle.**

2. An **increase in bone density** may also cause a reduction of the medullary canal, leading to an **aplastic anemia.**

3. Treatment

   —may include bone marrow transplantation for aplastic anemia.

D. Rickets

—results from a severe **deficiency of vitamin D.**

1. **Rickets is rare,** with most cases being secondary to some other underlying disease (i.e., renal dysfunction and gluten sensitivity).
2. This disease may **result in** bow legs with radiologic evidence of **flared metaphysis.**
3. The **cornerstone of treatment** is supplementation with vitamin D.

E. Osteoporosis

1. The **most common cause** of osteoporosis is **post-menopausal estrogen deprivation.**
2. **Diminished bone density leads** to pathologic fractures, especially in the **spine, femoral neck, and wrist.**
3. **Treatment** involves

   —**estrogen replacement.**

   —**calcium supplementation.**

   —**increasing activity** to maintain bone density.

VI. Bone Tumors

A. Metastatic disease

—is the **most common cause of malignant bone lesions.**

1. The **tumors that metastasize** most frequently include

   —breast.

   —prostate.

—thyroid.

—kidney.

—lung.

—adrenal.

a. **Tumor spread**

—is from direct invasion or via a hematogenous route.

b. **Spinal metastases**

—are through **Batson's venous plexus,** an alternative route of blood flow from the lower extremities to the heart that courses through the vertebral system.

2. **Evaluation**

a. **Plain films**

—are often unreliable.

b. **CT, MRI, and bone scans**

—are effective at demonstrating bone destruction.

c. **Metabolic** and **radiographic evaluation**

—should also be performed to identify the primary tumor.

d. **Biopsy of the metastatic bone lesion**

—is useful for confirming the diagnosis.

3. **Treatment**

—includes **internal fixation for impending fracture** (greater than 50% cortical involvement) followed by radiation therapy.

4. **Prognosis**

—Fifty percent of patients with pathologic fracture die of the disease within 3 months.

B. **Multiple myeloma**

—is the **most common primary malignancy of bone.**

1. This **disease occurs most commonly** in **men between 40–60 years of age.**

2. The **first symptom** is pain, especially **low back pain.**

3. **Evaluation**

a. **Laboratory evaluation** should include

—**serum protein electrophoresis.**

—**urinary protein analysis.**

b. **On urinalysis**

—Fifty percent of patients will have **Bence Jones** proteins.

c. A **plain radiographic survey**

—will show **diffuse osteolytic lesions.**

4. **Treatment**

a. **Chemotherapy** is used to treat systemic disease.

b. **Internal fixation** is necessary for impending fractures.

C. **Primary bone tumors**

—Characteristics of primary bone tumors are outlined in **Table 5-4.**

Table 5-4. Common Primary Bone Tumors

Tumor	Age (yrs)	Location	Evaluation	Treatment	Prognosis
Benign					
Osteoid osteoma	10–30	Lower extremities and spine	Plain film: sclerosis surrounding a radiolucent center (nidus); lesion < 1 cm	NSAIDs, resection	Excellent
Enchondroma	5–80	Appendicular skeleton, phalanges of fingers and toes most common	Plain film: lucent lesions with mineralization, "popcorn calcifications"	Observation, curettage and bone grafting	Good, propensity to differentiate into low-grade chondrosarcoma
Osteochondroma	< 20	Distal femur, humerus, and tibia	Plain film: outgrowth of cortical bone; pathology reveals cartilage cap	No treatment unless cosmetic deformity or pain secondary to local inflammation	Excellent
Chondroblastoma	10–40	Epiphysis of humerus, femur, and tibia	Plain film: osteolytic lesion with calcifications and thin sclerotic margin	Curettage and bone grafting; rare pulmonary metastasis treated with removal	Excellent
Nonossifying fibroma	<10	Metaphysis of long bones	Plain film: areas of translucency; incidental finding	Observation unless fracture requires curettage and bone grafting	Excellent
Fibrous dysplasia	<30	Craniofacial bones, femur, tibia, and ribs	Plain film: lucent lesion with "ground glass" appearance	Curettage and resection	Good, rare malignant transformation
Giant cell tumor	20–30	Epiphysis with extension into metaphysis (juxta-articular) of long bones	Plain film: lytic lesion with well defined borders and thinning of the cortex	Total resection with or without radiation therapy	Good but tumor has a 30% risk of recurrence and may metastasize

Malignant

Osteosarcoma	10–30	Metaphysis of the femur, tibia, and humerus	Plain film: cortical lucency with sclerosis, mineralized mass, and radiating spicules; CT or MRI best; Biopsy for confirmation	Irradiation ± chemotherapy followed by either limb sparing salvage or amputation	Depends on grade and stage of tumor
Chondrosarcoma	10–60	Pelvis, ribs, sternum, and femur	Plain film: destruction of bone with flecks of calcified tissue; Biopsy for confirmation	Limb sparing surgery or amputation	Depends on grade and stage of tumor
Fibrosarcoma	20–70	Femur, tibia, and humerus	Plain film: central lesion that expands to destroy cortex; Biopsy for confirmation	Amputation or resection and irradiation	35% 5-year survival
Ewing's sarcoma	5–15	Tibia, fibula, humerus, femur	Plain film: resemble osteomyelitis, "onion skin" layers in periosteum; biopsy for confirmation	Local irradiation and chemotherapy ± wide surgical resection	Often metastatic; 5-year survival about 50%

NSAIDs = nonsteroidal anti-inflammatory drugs.

Review Test

Directions: Each of the numbered items or incomplete statements in this section is followed by answers or by completions of the statement. Select the ONE lettered answer or completion that is BEST in each case.

1. A 20-year-old woman presents to the emergency room after having fallen from a window. She is awake, alert, and hemodynamically stable. She is complaining of right lower extremity pain and left wrist pain. Head and abdomen computed tomography (CT) scans and chest radiographs are negative. Radiographs reveal a distal radius fracture and a dislocated right hip. Which of the following is the most appropriate next step in the management of this patient?

(A) Perform CT scans of the hip and radius to define the injury
(B) Reduce the hip in the emergency room suite with conscious sedation
(C) Proceed immediately to the operating room for an open reduction of the hip
(D) Reduce the wrist first and then address the hip
(E) Place a femoral traction pin in the emergency room suite and place her in skeletal traction

2. A 19-year-old man was playing football when he felt a sudden pop in his right knee while avoiding a tackle. He developed an immediate effusion and pain with weight-bearing over the right knee. In the emergency room, radiographs were negative for fracture, and he was placed in a knee immobilizer and discharged. He now presents to the clinic with persistent pain and notes that his knee seems to "lock" at times. The swelling has improved and he has a positive McMurray's test, a negative posterior drawer, and a positive Lachman's test. Which of the following injuries is most likely present?

(A) Posterior cruciate ligament and meniscal tear
(B) Anterior and posterior cruciate ligament tear
(C) Anterior cruciate ligament and meniscal tear
(D) Isolated meniscal tear
(E) Patella fracture

3. A 16-year-old girl suffered an oblique distal femur fracture in a motorcycle accident and was treated with intramedullary nailing. The surgery was uncomplicated and took approximately 1.5 hours. The rest of the patient's evaluation, including head and abdominal computed tomography (CT) scans, was unremarkable. Twenty-four hours after leaving the operative suite, the nurse notes that the patient was breathing with difficulty. On evaluation, she is tachypneic, confused, and has small red lesions on her chest and back. Homans' sign is negative. Ultrasound of both lower extremities are negative. Which of the following is the most likely cause for this patient's decompensation?

(A) Pulmonary embolus from a calf deep vein thrombosis
(B) Unrecognized head injury
(C) Sepsis
(D) Fat emboli syndrome
(E) Alcohol withdrawal

4. A 75-year-old man presents to his primary care physician with complaints of right hip pain for the last 6 months. His doctor prescribed nonsteroidal anti-inflammatory drugs (NSAIDs), with no relief. There is now pain at night that wakes him from his sleep. His medical history is noncontributory, except for a long history of tobacco use. Radiographs reveal a lytic lesion in his femoral neck. Which of the following is the most likely diagnosis?

(A) Osteosarcoma
(B) Multiple myeloma
(C) Metastatic disease
(D) Chondrosarcoma
(E) Ewing's sarcoma

5. An orthopedic consult is requested in the neonatal intensive care unit for a premature infant with an obvious left clubfoot. Which of the following is the most appropriate initial treatment for this infant?

(A) Observation for resolution
(B) Passive stretching daily
(C) Immediate surgical correction when the patient is stable
(D) Serial casting with surgical correction after 6 months of age
(E) Wait for surgical correction until patient is ready to ambulate

6. As a result of a motorcycle accident, a 20-year-old healthy man suffers an open Grade I left midshaft displaced tibia fracture. The remainder of the trauma evaluation is negative. Which of the following is the best option for treating this patient?

(A) Irrigation of wound in the emergency room with closed reduction and casting
(B) Skeletal traction after irrigation in the emergency room
(C) Intravenous (IV) antibiotics and plastic surgery consult for wound coverage
(D) Immediate IV antibiotics with tetanus inoculation followed by irrigation of the wound in the emergency room
(E) Emergent wound irrigation and débridement with nailing of the tibia fracture in the operating room

7. An 85-year-old healthy woman who is an independent ambulator suffered a two-part minimally displaced left intertrochanteric hip fracture after a fall. She has no other injuries and is cleared from a medical standpoint. Which of the following is the best treatment option?

(A) Bed rest for 4–6 weeks until the pain resolves, and then protected weight bearing
(B) Skeletal traction for 4–6 weeks until healing occurs, and then crutch ambulating
(C) Open reduction and internal fixation and protected weight bearing for 4–6 weeks
(D) Total hip replacement
(E) Crutch ambulation for 4–6 weeks because this is a stable fracture

8. A 15-year-old boy presents to the clinic with left hip pain and a change in his gait. He is a healthy boy with no previous medical conditions. He has no history of recent trauma that he can remember. On physical examination he suffers from pain with range of motion of his left hip and walks with an antalgic gait. Anterior-posterior pelvis film shows an irregular epiphyseal plate. Which of the following is the most appropriate treatment measure for this patient?

(A) Hip spica cast for 6–8 months
(B) Restricted weight bearing and observation
(C) Operative placement of bone graft
(D) Bed rest with abduction pillow
(E) Surgical pinning of epiphysis

Answers and Explanations

1-B. This patient is stable and has no life-threatening injuries, so her orthopedic injuries can be addressed. A dislocated hip is an orthopedic emergency and must be addressed quickly. Conscious sedation with reduction of the hip in the emergency room is generally the preferred method of treatment. Open reduction is reserved after multiple attempts at closed reduction have failed. Timely reduction reduces the risk of avascular necrosis of the femoral head and subsequent post-traumatic degenerative osteoarthritis. Skeletal traction may be necessary if the hip remains unstable after reduction, as may be seen in the presence of an associated acetabular fracture. Computed tomography (CT) scans would not provide additional information that would alter the initial management of this patient.

2-C. This patient most likely suffered an anterior cruciate ligament (ACL) and a meniscal tear. The Lachman's test flexes the knee to 30° and tests the anterior displacement of the tibia on the femur. This is the most sensitive test for a tear in the ACL. The McMurray's test is used for meniscal tears. A symptom of locking is suggestive for meniscal tear. Treatment includes arthroscopy for débridement or repair of the meniscus and ACL reconstruction. A negative posterior drawer sign helps to rule out a posterior cruciate ligament tear. A patellar fracture would not generally be associated with the physical findings found.

3-D. This patient has most likely developed fat emboli syndrome. This commonly is the result of the infusion of fat from the marrow of a broken long bone, especially the femur, into the bloodstream.

The classic triad (Bergman's triad) for fat emboli syndrome is dyspnea, petechiae, and mental status changes. Treatment is supportive until the symptoms resolve. In severe cases acute respiratory distress syndrome may develop. Homans' sign, which tests for calf pain in the presence of a calf deep venous thrombosis, was negative, and the ultrasound of the lower extremities was also negative, making a pulmonary embolus from a lower extremity thrombosis unlikely. Sepsis is unlikely because the fracture was not open and other signs (i.e., fever, hypotension) are not present. Head injuries presenting at this point in the hospital course would be unlikely in the setting of a normal head computed tomography (CT) scan. Symptoms of alcohol withdrawal generally do not present this early during a patient's hospital course.

4-C. The most common cause of a malignant bone tumor is metastatic carcinoma. This patient most likely suffers from an undiagnosed primary lung cancer. Further evaluation should include computed tomography (CT) scans of the chest, abdomen, and pelvis. Also, blood work to include complete blood count with differential and blood chemistry should also be performed. Bone scan is helpful in finding other skeletal lesions. CT, magnetic resonance imaging (MRI), or biopsy of the lesion can be used to further define the lesion. For a metastatic femoral neck lesion that is an impending fracture, the treatment is internal fixation. Osteosarcoma is seen in a younger population. Chondrosarcoma may be seen in this age group, but the diagnosis will be made with the radiographic evaluation and biopsy. Ewing's sarcoma is seen in children and adolescents. Multiple myeloma is diagnosed with serum protein electrophoresis and a bone survey. Metastatic disease occurs much more commonly in primary bone tumors.

5-D. Clubfoot is best initially treated with serial casting every 1 to 2 weeks with gradual molding to improve the deformity. If the clubfoot is rigid, casting may provide minimal improvement. Surgery should be performed after 6 months of age if the deformity persists despite serial casting. Observation alone and passive stretching would be inadequate therapies. Immediate surgical correction is unnecessary, although delaying surgery until the patient is ambulating would also be inappropriate.

6-E. This patient has an open tibia fracture, and this is a surgical emergency. To decrease the chances of an infection, surgical débridement of all devitalized tissue and irrigation of the wound should be performed within 6–8 hours after the injury. Such extensive irrigation and débridement should be performed in the operating room and not in the emergency room. Grade I/II open tibia fractures can be treated with intramedullary nail fixation after irrigation and débridement. Grade III fractures require external fixation and possible plastic surgery consult for wound coverage. Intravenous (IV) antibiotics and tetanus are necessary in all open fractures. The patient should undergo a repeat washout in the operating room 48–72 hours after initial treatment. IV antibiotics and wound coverage without adequate débridement would be inadequate treatment.

7-C. The best treatment for an independent ambulator is open reduction and internal fixation (ORIF). Bed rest is associated with multiple complications including decubitus ulcers, pneumonia, deep venous thrombosis, and pulmonary edema. ORIF provides pain control from stabilization of the bone and early protected ambulating. Nonoperative treatment for proximal femur fracture is only indicated in patients who are not operative candidates secondary to their medical problems. Pin fixation of the hip is adequate without the need for a total hip replacement.

8-E. This patient suffers from a slipped capital femoral epiphysis. This most commonly occurs in adolescent African-American boys between the ages of 12 and 15. They present with hip pain and change in their gait. They are at significant risk for avascular necrosis of the femoral head. The only effective treatment to prevent this complication and to prevent further slippage is to surgically place a pin to fix the epiphysis. Bed rest, observation, and spica casting would be inadequate treatment measures in this patient. Surgical pinning is adequate treatment without the need for bone grafting.

6

Urology

Terence N. Chapman, Brant R. Fulmer, Victor M. Brugh III

I. Functional Anatomy of the Genitourinary System (Figure 6.1)

A. Kidneys

1. **The kidneys receive** 20% of cardiac output via a **single renal artery** in 75% of patients.

2. **Venous drainage** is via the renal veins into the vena cava.

   —The renal veins run **anterior** to the renal arteries.

3. The kidneys are **innervated by the renal plexus,** which exerts **vasomotor** control.

B. Bladder

1. **Innervation** is from S2–S4 segments.

2. **Blood supply** derives mainly from **superior** and **inferior vesical arteries,** which are branches of the hypogastric artery.

C. Prostate gland (Figure 6.2) and seminal vesicles

1. The **prostate gland**

   —is a 20 g, **walnut-shaped organ** situated at the bladder neck.

   —is responsible for approximately 20% of seminal fluid production.

   —is divided into anatomic zones (see Figure 6-2).

2. **The seminal vesicles**

   —are paired structures, which secrete a fructose-rich fluid comprising 60% of the ejaculatory fluid, then empty through the ejaculatory ducts in the prostatic urethra.

3. **Blood supply**

   —derives from the inferior vesical and prostatic arteries.

   —is **rich in α_1-adrenergic receptors.**

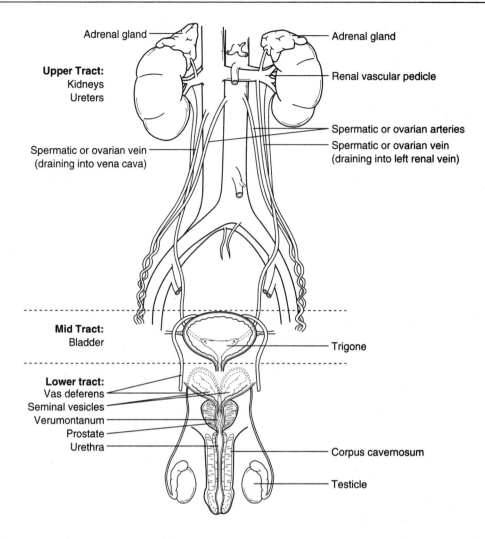

Figure 6.1. The genitourinary system.

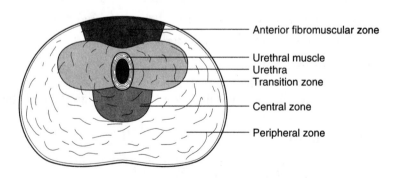

Figure 6.2. Cross-section of the prostate gland.

D. Penis (Figure 6.3) and urethra

1. Arterial supply to the penis

—is derived mainly from the (paired) internal pudendal arteries, which are branches of the internal iliac artery.

2. Each pudendal artery becomes the penile artery and gives off 3 branches.

a. The **dorsal artery** controls tumescence of glans penis.

b. The **bulbourethral artery** supplies the corpus spongiosum, which contains the urethra.

c. The **cavernous arteries** are responsible for engorgement of the interconnected corpora cavernosa.

3. Skin and superficial penile structures drain into the saphenous system.

—Deeper structures drain to **the deep dorsal** and **internal pudendal veins.**

4. The cavernous nerves arise from parasympathetic (S2–S4) and sympathetic (T10–12) nerves via the pelvic plexus.

—They are responsible for primary neural control of erection (parasympathetic) and detumescence (sympathetic).

E. Scrotum and testes

1. The scrotum maintains testicular temperature

—at the optimal 2° C below core body temperature for spermatogenesis.

2. Three arteries supply the testis:

—testicular

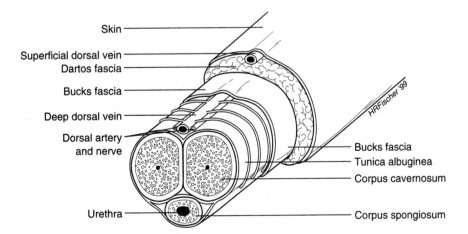

Figure 6.3. The penis. (Adapted with permission from Lawrence PF: *Essentials of Surgical Specialties.* Baltimore, Williams & Wilkins, 1993, p 377.)

—**cremasteric**

—**artery to the vas deferens**

3. **Each testis is sheathed in tunica albuginea**

   —limiting expansion in cases of inflammation (e.g., mumps orchitis).

4. **Gonadal veins drain** into the **vena cava (on the right)** and the **renal vein (on the left).**

5. **Varicocele**

   —is the **engorgement of the pampiniform plexus of veins in the scrotum.**

   —results from retrograde venous flow.

   —is common on left side owing to venous anatomy.

   —**Varicoceles** that do not reduce in the supine position suggest retroperitoneal or renal malignancy, especially on the left side.

II. Infections of the Genitourinary Tract

A. **General terms and definitions**

1. **Bacteriuria**

   —is the presence of bacteria in the urine.

2. **Pyuria**

   —is the presence of leukocytes (white blood cells) in the urine.

3. **Urinary tract infection (UTI)**

   a. **Uncomplicated UTI**

      —refers to an infection in a patient with a structurally and functionally normal urinary tract.

   b. **Complicated UTI**

      —refers to an infection in a patient with pyelonephritis or a structural or functional abnormality of the urinary tract.

4. **Pyelonephritis**

   a. **Acute pyelonephritis**

      —is the clinical syndrome of fever and flank pain accompanied by bacteriuria and pyuria.

   b. **Chronic pyelonephritis**

      —refers to an atrophic, scarred kidney from repeated infection.

      —The diagnosis is made on the basis of history and radiologic findings.

B. **Risk factors** include

   —**female gender** secondary to decreased urethral length.

   —hospitalization and **catheterization.**

   —concurrent disease.

   —history of UTI.

—urologic anatomic abnormality (e.g., vesicoureteral reflux).

C. Pathogenesis

1. **Most infections ascend** from the lower urinary tract, although hematogenous spread may rarely be the source of infection.

2. **Pathogens** are usually from the **fecal reservoir** or other enteric origin.

   a. The **most common bacterial cause** of UTI is *Escherichia coli* (90%).

   b. **Other bacterial species** include
      —*Staphylococcus.*
      —*Proteus.*
      —*Klebsiella.*
      —*Enterococcus.*
      —*Pseudomonas.*

   c. **Risk factors** for **fungal infection** (*Candida albicans* most common) include
      —**diabetes.**
      —prolonged catheterization.
      —extended hospitalization.
      —immunosuppression.

   d. **Adenovirus**
      —While rare in adults, adenovirus can cause hemorrhagic cystitis in children.

D. Presentation

1. **Cystitis**

   —usually presents with **dysuria, urgency, and frequency.**
   —Fever and suprapubic pain may rarely be present.

2. **Pyelonephritis**

   —classically presents with the triad of **fever, flank pain, and pyuria.**

E. Diagnosis

1. **Urinalysis**

   —will often reveal hematuria and may be positive for leukocyte esterase and nitrite.

2. **Microscopic examination of the urine**

   —usually reveals white blood cells, red blood cells, and bacteria.

3. **Urine culture and sensitivity**

   —is an essential diagnostic component.

   a. **Colony counts higher than 10^5 per mL** are considered diagnostic in all patients.

   b. **Colony counts lower than 10^5 per mL** may be considered diagnostic in symptomatic patients.

F. Treatment

1. **Uncomplicated UTIs**

—may be treated with short-course (1–5 days) of oral antibiotic therapy.

2. Complicated UTIs

—often require a longer course (14–21 days) of antibiotic therapy, with a variable period of parenteral antibiotics.

G. Complications

1. Urosepsis

—can result from severe pyelonephritis.

2. A perinephric or intrarenal abscess

—should be suspected when 48–72 hours of appropriate antibiotic therapy fails to result in clinical improvement.

—often requires open or percutaneous drainage.

3. Urolithiasis

—can result from urease-producing organisms such as *Proteus* species.

4. Papillary necrosis

—can result in sloughing of renal papillae and ureteral obstruction, and is most commonly seen in patients with diabetes.

H. Other infections of the genitourinary tract

1. Urethritis

—caused by *Neisseria gonorrhoeae* or *Chlamydia trachomatis* should be suspected in sexually active patients with dysuria and urethral discharge.

2. Acute epididymitis

—may be caused by similar organisms as in urethritis.

—is associated with **acute severe pain and swelling of the epididymis.**

3. Mumps orchitis

a. Although rare, mumps orchitis may present as a swollen, tender testicle typically 3–4 days after parotitis in adult men.

b. Impaired spermatogenesis may result.

4. Prostatitis

a. Acute bacterial prostatitis

—is an acute inflammation of the prostate commonly caused by gram-negative (*E. coli, Proteus*) organisms.

—requires antibiotic therapy.

—Patients can be quite ill and rectal examinations can incite bacteremia.

b. Chronic prostatitis

—is characterized by inflammation that can be caused by chronic bacterial infection.

—The inflammation may also be present without evidence of infection.

c. Prostatodynia

—describes a syndrome of chronic prostatic and pelvic pain with a pathologically normal prostate gland.

III. Urolithiasis

A. Epidemiology

1. Urolithiasis is more likely to affect **men.**

   —The male to female ratio is 3:1.

2. Peak incidence is 20–40 years of age.

3. Urolithiasis is more common in patients living in warmer, drier climates (e.g., Southeast United States).

4. In the United States, the peak months for stone formation are July, August, and September.

B. Risk factors include

—low water intake and diets high in stone-promoting substances (e.g., oxalate, protein).

—hereditary factors (e.g., cystinuria).

C. Urinary calculi

—Types and causes of these calculi are listed in **Table 6-1.**

D. Diagnosis

Table 6-1. Types and Causes of Urinary Calculi

Major Type	Etiologies
Calcium stones (80%–85%)	**Absorptive hypercalciuria:** Increased intestinal absorption of calcium **Resorptive hypercalciuria:** Associated with hyperparathyroidism **Renal hypercalciuria:** Primary renal defect resulting in increased tubular secretion of calcium **Hyperoxaluria:** Ca^{2+}-oxalate stones resulting from steatorrhea, causing calcium binding to fat over oxalate and leading to increased absorption and urinary excretion of oxalate **Hypocitraturia:** Associated with renal tubular acidosis (Type 1), thiazide therapy, and fasting; urinary citrate normally inhibits stone formation
Uric acid stones (< 5%)	Low urine pH results in uric acid precipitation; may be associated with gout and myeloproliferative disorders but most patients do not have elevated serum uric acid levels; urine pH usually < 5.5
Cystine stones	Congenital metabolic defect in renal absorption of cystine resulting in cystinuria and formation of extremely hard stones
Infection stones	Infection with urea-splitting organisms (e.g., *Proteus*) causes increased urinary pH, precipitating magnesium ammonium phosphate (**struvite**) stones

1. The **most common presenting findings** include **flank pain and hematuria.**

2. **Laboratory studies**

   —should include urinalysis, white blood cell count, and creatinine.

3. **Imaging studies**

   a. **Plain radiograph (kidney, ureters, bladder, or KUB) and a tomography scan**

      —are useful initial studies to identify radiopaque calculi such as calcium stones.

      —Plain radiographs do not give information about the degree of obstruction or presence of radiolucent calculi, such as uric acid stones.

   b. **Ultrasound**

      —is often useful to determine obstruction, stone size, and location.

   c. **Intravenous pyelography (IVP)**

      —is useful for assessment of the anatomy of collecting system, excretion, and obstruction.

   d. **Spiral computed tomography (CT) scanning without contrast**

      —is very sensitive and specific for urinary calculi, because **nearly all stones are radiopaque on CT.**

4. **Patients with recurrent or complicated urolithiasis**

   —should undergo evaluation for potential contributing metabolic factors.

   a. Perform a **24-hour urine analysis to** determine the urine levels of

      —calcium.

      —phosphate.

      —uric acid.

      —magnesium.

      —oxalate.

      —citrate.

      —sodium.

      —potassium.

      —creatinine.

   b. Identify **other disease states** that predispose the patient to stone formation (e.g., inflammatory bowel disease, and oxalate stones).

   c. Rule out **hyperparathyroidism,** especially in younger female patients with multiple stone episodes.

      —**Serum calcium** is a useful screening test for hyperparathyroidism.

E. **Treatment**

   1. **Medical management**

      a. **Fluid administration**

         —is the mainstay of therapy for all types of urinary calculus disease and should approach 2–3 L daily.

      b. **Dietary restriction**

         —is only useful in patients with a history of increased intake of specific substances (e.g., oxalate-rich foods such as coffee, tea, and chocolate).

—**Calcium restriction** may actually worsen stone disease.

c. Alkalinization of the urine

—with agents such as potassium citrate raise urinary pH and citrate, a stone inhibitor which complexes calcium in solution. Elevated pH levels inhibit uric acid stone formation.

d. Gastrointestinal absorption inhibitor therapy

—with agents such as cellulose phosphate bind calcium in the gut and prevent absorption (i.e., absorptive hypercalciuria).

e. Thiazide diuretics

—correct "renal leak" hypercalciuria by reducing urinary calcium excretion, thereby decreasing stone formation.

f. Allopurinol (a xanthine oxidase inhibitor)

—reduces both serum and urinary uric acid levels.

2. Surgical management

a. Indications for emergent surgical intervention in patients with urolithiasis include

—fever.

—UTI (especially in patients with diabetes).

—solitary kidney.

b. Relative indications for surgical management include intractable symptoms such as

—renal insufficieny.

—pain.

—prolonged obstruction.

—chronic infection.

c. Different types of surgical intervention

—are outlined in **Table 6-2.**

IV. Neoplasms of the Genitourinary Tract

A. Benign prostatic hyperplasia (BPH)

1. Pathogenesis and presentation

a. BPH arises

—from age- and androgen-dependent hyperplasia of periurethral glands and stroma in the **transition zone** of the prostate (see Figure 6-2).

b. Symptoms

(1) Irritative symptoms

—(e.g., nocturia, frequency and dysuria) result from hypertrophy-induced bladder instability in response to chronic obstruction.

(2) Obstructive symptoms

—(e.g., hesitancy, decreased force of stream, urinary retention) result from urethral compression by adenomatous tissue.

Table 6-2. Surgical Options for Urolithiasis

Procedure	Method
Percutaneous nephrostomy	Percutaneous placement of tube into renal pelvis to provide rapid relief of obstruction
Ureteral stent placement	Retrograde passage of stent to relieve obstruction and passively dilate the ureter to allow for stone passage
Shock Wave Lithotripsy (SWL)	Stone fragmentation via shock waves focused on the stone using ultrasound or fluoroscopic localization
Retrograde ureteroscopy	Stone removal or fragmentation under direct visualization using a fiberoptic scope via a retrograde, transurethral approach
Percutaneous fragmentation	Direct stone fragmentation through percutaneously placed nephrostomy tubes
Nephrolithotomy/ ureterolithotomy	Open surgical removal of stones

(3) Other signs and symptoms may include

—hematuria (gross or microscopic).

—recurrent UTIs.

—renal insufficiency.

  2. Diagnosis

   a. A **digital rectal examination** estimates

—gland size.

—consistency and presence of possible malignancy (i.e., nodularity or induration).

   b. A **palpable bladder**

—may be found in patients with significant **urinary retention.**

   c. Symptoms of BPH

—are quantified using the American Urological Association (AUA) symptom questionnaire, a series of 7 questions, with each ranking 0–5, for a total possible score of 35.

—Patients may be grouped into mild, moderate, or severe categories, with therapy often guided by symptom severity.

   d. Uroflowmetry

—is often used to objectively assess rate of flow; however, obstruction cannot be diagnosed solely with this test.

  3. Treatment

   a. Medical therapy

—has become the first line of treatment for most men with mild to moderate BPH.

   (1) α_1-Adrenergic antagonists (e.g., doxazosin)

—decrease smooth muscle tone at the bladder neck and prostate capsule, thus reducing obstruction.

(2) 5α-Reductase inhibitors (e.g., finasteride)

—have been shown to shrink the prostate gland over a period of months and may decrease prostatic bleeding episodes.

—**block the conversion of testosterone to its more potent metabolite, dihydrotestosterone (DHT).**

b. Surgical removal of the obstructive tissue

—can be accomplished in many ways, varying according to the individual patient.

—is usually reserved for severe symptoms.

(1) Transurethral resection of the prostate (TURP) is the gold standard of therapy for BPH.

(2) Absolute indications for TURP include

—renal insufficiency.

—bladder calculi.

—recurrent urinary retention.

—UTIs.

—gross hematuria.

(3) "Transurethral resection (TUR) syndrome"

—is a complication of TURP caused by dilutional **hyponatremia and cerebral edema** related to massive exchange of water through venous channels in the prostate.

(a) Glycine solution, as a TURP irrigant, has been implicated in cases of hyperammonemia and mental status changes.

(b) Treatment involves diuresis and careful correction of serum sodium.

(4) Other procedures

(a) Open prostatectomy involves simple enucleation of the adenoma and is usually reserved for glands weighing 80 g or more. It involves "shelling out" only the adenomatous tissue (in contrast to radical prostatectomy).

(b) Laser ablation of the prostate substitutes laser energy for electrocautery and provides excellent hemostasis.

(c) Microwave thermotherapy and **transurethral needle ablation** (TUNA) are newer modalities that utilize microwave and radiofrequency energy to destroy prostatic tissue.

(d) Urethral stents may be used in patients too ill for other procedures.

B. Prostate cancer

1. Epidemiology

a. Adenocarcinoma of the prostate is the most prevalent cancer in **men.**

b. Prostate cancer is **more common** and associated with a higher mortality in **African-Americans** for unclear reasons.

2. Pathogenesis

—**Prostate cancer arises** from the **peripheral zone glandular**

epithelium in **70%** of cases, **transition zone** in 15%, and the **central zone** in 15%.

3. **Diagnosis**
   a. A **digital rectal examination** is used
      —for cancer detection.
      —to estimate the degree of local spread.
   b. The **prostate-specific antigen (PSA) level**
      —is a key parameter in the evaluation and diagnosis of prostate cancer.
      (1) A **PSA level** of **4.0 ng/mL** is considered the upper limit of normal.
      (2) The **rate of PSA change over time (PSA velocity)** and **free (unbound) PSA** may be clinically useful in addition to the total PSA in certain cases.
      (3) The PSA level and Gleason tumor grade (see IV B 4) are predictive of the **stage** of prostate cancer.
      (4) Poorly differentiated cancers may not produce PSA.
      (5) **PSA may also be elevated in cases of BPH, prostatitis, and chronic catheterization.**
   c. **Ultrasound-guided biopsy**
      —allows zone-directed sampling of the prostate and is the primary method of diagnosis.
   d. **Chest radiograph and radionuclide bone scanning**
      —are used to assess for metastatic disease.
      —Most metastatic bone lesions are **osteoblastic** on plain radiograph.
   e. **CT scan of the pelvis**
      —is used to identify adenopathy or extraprostatic disease.

4. **Staging and grading of prostate cancer**
   —is presented in **Table 6-3.**
   a. Pelvic (obturator) **lymph node dissection** is performed to stage the cancer.
   b. **Tumors are graded** from 2–10 on the **Gleason grading system,** in which the grades of the two most representative portions are combined into one **sum** (e.g., Gleason 3 + 3 = 6).

5. **Treatment**
   a. **Treatment is directed** by many factors including
      —presence or absence of extraprostatic or distant disease.
      —patient preference.
      —age and performance status.
   b. **For cancer limited to the prostate** (T1a–c, T2a–b), **radical prostatectomy is often curative.**
      (1) Associated complications may include **impotence and incontinence.**
      (2) This is generally offered to patients with a minimum 10-year life expectancy.
   c. **External beam radiation (XRT)**
      —is often combined with hormonal deprivation therapy.

Table 6-3. Staging System for Adenocarcinoma of the Prostate*

Tumor, Node, Metastasis (TNM) Stage	Description
Tumor	
T1	Tumor found incidentally (e.g., after TURP)
T1a	< 5% of TURP specimen
T1b	> 5% of TURP specimen
T1c	Discovered at biopsy for an elevated PSA only
T2	Tumor confined to the prostate
T2a	One lobe
T2b	Both lobes
T3	Tumor extends through the prostate capsule
T3a	Unilateral or bilateral
T3b	Seminal vesicle
T4	Tumor is fixed to or invades adjacent structures
Node	
N1	Single lymph node < 2 cm
N2	Single lymph node 2–5 cm Multiple lymph nodes < 5 cm
N3	Lymph node(s) > 5 cm
Metastasis	
M1	Distant metastases

*1997 UICC Staging
TURP = transurethral resection of the prostate; PSA = prostate-specific antigen.

—is less commonly used as monotherapy.

—10-year survival is similar to radical prostatectomy.

d. **Interstitial brachytherapy with or without external beam "boost"**

—is offered to patients with low clinical stage (T1–T2) cancers.

—has shown early promising results in the treatment of lower and moderate grade tumors.

e. **Watchful waiting** may play a role

—in low-grade, low stage cancers.

—in a patient of advanced age or with other significant morbidities.

    f. Locally advanced disease (T3)

      —may be treated with XRT after radical prostatectomy (i.e., for positive margins).

    g. Metastatic disease

      —can be successfully palliated by androgen deprivation or local radiation in cases of symptomatic bony lesions.

      (1) Bilateral orchiectomy is the most cost-effective form of **androgen deprivation.**

      (2) Luteinizing hormone-releasing hormone (LHRH) agonists (e.g., leuprolide) inhibit androgen production in the testes by central inhibition of luteinizing hormone release.

      (3) Ketoconazole (an antifungal and cytochrome p450 inhibitor) causes rapid lowering of testosterone to castrate levels (e.g., spinal cord compression or bilateral ureteral obstruction).

      (4) Palliative radiotherapy may be used for **bone pain** or spinal compression.

      (5) Combination chemotherapy (e.g., paclitaxel and estramustine) is reserved for late metastatic disease that has "escaped" hormonal deprivation.

C. Renal cell carcinoma (RCC)

  1. The **only firmly established risk factor** for RCC is **smoking.**

  2. Pathology and differential diagnosis

    a. RCC originates from proximal tubular epithelium and is typically highly **vascular tumors.**

    b. Renal "adenomas"

      —are considered by many pathologists to be likely small RCCs.

    c. Oncocytomas

      —are treated clinically like RCCs.

      —are characterized radiographically by spoke-wheel vessels and a central stellate scar.

      —Their malignant potential is controversial.

    d. Angiomyolipomas

      —are hamartomas seen sporadically or in syndromes such as tuberous sclerosis.

      —Large lesions (bigger than 4 cm) may require excision or embolization if symptomatic (e.g., pain, bleeding).

  3. Diagnosis

    a. The **triad of flank pain, an abdominal mass, and hematuria** is seen in only 10% of cases.

    b. Most patients present with **gross or microscopic hematuria.**

    c. One third of patients present with metastatic disease (e.g., lung, liver, bone, adrenal, and contralateral kidney disease).

    d. von Hippel-Lindau syndrome is associated with

      —multifocal and recurrent RCCs.

      —renal cysts.

      —central nervous system (cerebellar) tumors.

—pheochromocytomas.

e. **CT scanning with contrast (Figure 6.4)**

—is the cornerstone of diagnosis.

—typically reveals an enhancing solid or cystic renal mass.

f. **Angiography**

—may be used in the setting of planned partial nephrectomy, abnormal anatomy ("horseshoe kidney"), or hypervascularity.

4. **Paraneoplastic syndromes**

—associated with RCCs are outlined in **Table 6-4.**

5. **Staging**

—of RCC is outlined in **Table 6-5.**

6. **Treatment**

a. **Radical nephrectomy**

—with or without removal of the adrenal gland and occasionally tumor thrombus in the renal vein or inferior vena cava is the standard treatment of RCC.

b. **Partial ("nephron-sparing") nephrectomy**

—is used in cases where radical nephrectomy would result in dialysis dependence.

—is gaining wider popularity for smaller, peripheral lesions, in otherwise healthy patients.

c. **Embolization** is usually reserved for

—large tumors to facilitate surgical removal.

—palliation and control of hemorrhage in advanced cases.

d. **Immunotherapy with interleukin (IL)-2 administration**

—to stimulate lymphocytes is an investigational therapy for certain cases of metastatic RCC.

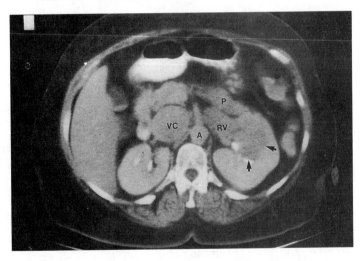

Figure 6.4. Computed tomography (CT) scan of a renal cell carcinoma (RCC). Note the mass in the left kidney (*arrows*) with extension into the renal vein (RV) and into the inferior vena cava (VC), which is enlarged. A = aorta; P = pancreas. (Reprinted with permission from Daffner RH: *Clinical Radiology, The Essentials,* 2nd ed. Baltimore, Lippincott Williams & Wilkins, 1999, p 348.)

Table 6-4. Paraneoplastic Syndromes Associated With Renal Cell Carcinoma (RCC)

Clinical Finding	Causative Hormone Secreted by Tumor
Erythrocytosis	Erythropoietin
Hypercalcemia	Parathyroid hormone (PTH)-like protein
Cushing's syndrome	Adrenocorticotropic hormone (ACTH)
Hypoglycemia	Insulin
Hepatic dysfunction (Stauffer's syndrome)	Unknown (reversible after nephrectomy)

    D. Transitional cell carcinoma

        1. Overview

            a. These **tumors most commonly affect** the **bladder.**

                —They may also affect the renal pelvis and ureter.

            b. Transitional cell carcinoma occurs at a male to female ratio of nearly 3:1.

        2. Risk factors include

            —**cigarette smoking (major cause).**

            —working with rubber and aniline dye.

            —exposure to cyclophosphamide.

Table 6-5. Staging of Renal Cell Carcinoma (RCC)

Tumor, Node, Metastasis (TNM) Staging	Description
Tumor	
T1	Tumor < 7.0 cm (confined to kidney)
T2	Tumor > 7.0 cm (confined to kidney)
T3a	Adrenal or perinephric fat invasion within Gerota's fascia
T3b	Renal vein or caval extension below diaphragm
T3c	Caval extension above diaphragm
Node	
N1	Solitary node
N2	Multiple nodes
Metastasis	
M1	Distant metastases

3. **Pathogenesis**
   a. **Most cancers in the bladder** arise from **transitional epithelium.**
   b. **Squamous cell carcinoma**
      —is associated with **schistosomiasis** (bilharzia); however, it is also associated with chronic irritation (e.g., foreign bodies, calculi).
   c. **Adenocarcinoma**
      —is rare and usually associated with embryologic defects (e.g., urachal remnant and bladder exstrophy).

4. **Diagnosis**
   a. An **IVP**
      —performed in the setting of **hematuria** (gross or microscopic) often reveals filling defects in the bladder, renal pelvis, or ureter.
   b. **Cystoscopy**
      —can identify small tumors and carcinoma in situ in the bladder.
   c. **Retrograde urography**
      —can more precisely define upper tract tumors.
   d. **Ureteroscopy**
      —allows visualization and biopsy of upper tract lesions.
   e. **Voided urine cytology**
      —can provide additional evidence of malignancy.

5. **Staging**

   —of transitional cell carcinoma is outlined in **Table 6-6.**

Table 6-6. Staging of Transitional Cell Carcinoma of the Bladder

Tumor, Node, Metastasis (TNM) Staging	Description
Tumor	
Tis (cis)	Carcinoma in situ
T1	Invades lamina propria
T2	Invades muscle
T3	Invades perivesical fat
T4	Invades adjacent organs
Node	
N1	One node < 2 cm
N2	2 cm < node(s) < 5 cm
N3	Node > 5 cm
Metastasis	
M1	Distant metastases

a. **Transurethral resection or biopsy**

—**requires a specimen containing bladder muscle** to determine the presence of invasion.

b. **Bimanual examination**

—after resection is used to assess for residual mass.

c. **CT scanning and chest radiography**

—assess for metastatic disease.

6. **Treatment** of **localized lesions**

a. **Transurethral resection**

—can be used to treat **superficial lesions** (Ta, T1).

—Close follow-up is required because **recurrence is common** (70%).

b. **Radical cystectomy**

—with urinary diversion is used when **muscle invasion** (T2, T3) **by the tumor is present** on biopsy specimen.

—**Combined chemotherapy and radiation** is an alternative to cystectomy in certain cases.

c. **Nephroureterectomy**

—including a cuff of bladder surrounding the ureteral orifice *en bloc,* is the standard treatment for **renal pelvic or ureteral transitional cell tumors.**

d. **Bacille Calmette-Guérin (BCG) vaccine**

—instilled intravesically induces an immune response that may cause **regression of superficial lesions** (T1 and Tis).

e. **Combination chemotherapy**

—is used to treat **metastatic disease,** which confers a poor prognosis (20% 2-year survival).

E. **Testicular cancer (Table 6-7)**

1. **Epidemiology and risk factors**

a. **Testicular cancer generally affects** men in the third and fourth decades.

b. **Risk factors** include

—cryptorchidism.

—white race.

—high socioeconomic class.

2. **Pathogenesis**

a. Approximately **2.5%** of testicular cancers may be **bilateral.**

b. **Germ cell tumors** account for more than 90% of testis tumors.

(1) **Seminomas** account for **35%** of germ cell tumors.

(2) **Nonseminomatous germ cell tumors (NSGCT)** refer to all other histologies, **even if mixed with seminoma in any proportion.**

c. **Nongerm cell tumors** include

—lymphomas (seen in older men).

—Leydig and Sertoli cell tumors.

Table 6-7. Seminomatous Versus Nonseminomatous Germ Cell Tumors of the Testes

Germ Cell Tumor	Tumor Markers	Treatment	Cure Rates
Seminomatous (35%)	β-HCG: in 7% of lesions	**Low stage:** Radical inguinal orchiectomy and retroperitoneal radiation	More than 90% with low stage surgically resectable disease
	AFP: never	**High stage:** Preoperative platinum-based chemotherapy and surgical excision of residual mass	Approximately 75% with high stage disease treated with primary chemotherapy
Nonseminomatous Embryonal cell carcinoma (20%)	AFP ± β-HCG frequently (70%) elevated	**Low stage:** Radical inguinal orchiectomy and retroperitoneal lymph node dissection	More than 90% with low stage surgically resectable disease
Teratoma (5%)			
Choriocarcinoma (< 1%)			
Yolk-sac tumors (rare)		**High stage:** Preoperative chemotherapy and surgical excision of residual mass	High stage disease associated with 60%–80% 5-year survival

β-HCG = beta-human chorionic gonadotropin; AFP = α-fetoprotein.

        —gonadoblastomas.

        —sarcomas.

  3. Diagnosis

    a. The **classic presentation** is that of a **painless, hard, testicular mass.**

      (1) Masses in the testicle are malignant until proven otherwise.

      (2) Intrascrotal, nontesticular masses are predominantly benign.

    b. Occasionally patients present with palpable abdominal disease.

    c. The **presence of an α-fetoprotein (AFP) level rules out pure seminoma.**

    d. Lactate dehydrogenase (LDH) levels correlate with tumor bulk.

    e. Ultrasound

      —is useful to confirm position of a mass in the testis and thus to differentiate it from benign processes.

    f. Chest radiograph

      —can identify pulmonary metastases

    g. CT scan

      —quantifies retroperitoneal and mediastinal tumor burden.

4. Treatment of testis tumors

—is primarily by **radical inguinal orchiectomy,** avoiding scrotal violation at all costs, to avoid interruption of lymphatic channels.

—Further therapy is dictated by the stage of the disease, (i.e., metastases to retroperitoneal lymph nodes or distant organs) [see Table 6-7] and is mainly chemotherapy with or without surgery.

V. Trauma

A. Renal trauma

1. Classification of renal injuries is based on the

—**size of the injury.**

—**stability** of the injury (e.g., expanding hematoma).

—**presence or absence of urinary extravasation.**

—**extent of involvement of the renal artery and vein.**

2. Evaluation

a. Hematuria may be absent in 10%–25% of renal injuries.

—The amount of blood may not reflect the severity of the injury.

b. A **CT scan** will identify

—urinary extravasation.

—parenchymal lacerations.

—hematomas.

—devascularization.

c. IVP

—identifies whether both kidneys function.

d. Nonvisualization during IVP may be secondary to

—congenital absence of kidney.

—shock.

—renal artery thrombosis or avulsion.

—high-grade obstruction.

—ectopia.

e. Arteriography may be indicated with nonvisualized kidneys on IVP or nonenhancing kidney on CT.

—This allows for identification of renal artery thrombosis or avulsion.

3. Indications for surgical exploration include

—**uncontrolled bleeding with hemodynamic instability.**

—**renovascular injury.**

—**penetrating injury to the kidney or flank.**

—**major urinary extravasation.**

—Many surgeons prefer isolation of renal pedicle before exploration.

B. Bladder and urethral trauma

1. These injuries

—may be associated with both blunt and penetrating trauma.

—are frequently associated with **pelvic fractures.**

2. **Evaluation**
   a. Over **95% will have hematuria** on urinalysis.
   b. **Blood at the urethral meatus or a "high riding" prostate** on rectal examination are highly suggestive of a urethral injury.
   c. A **retrograde cystourethrogram** should be performed if such an injury is suspected.

3. **Treatment**
   a. **Intraperitoneal bladder rupture**
      —requires **surgical exploration and repair.**
   b. **Extraperitoneal bladder rupture**
      —with minimal extravasation may be managed with urethral catheter drainage, although severe extravasation warrants surgical repair.
   c. **Urethral injuries without extravasation**
      —can be treated with **urethral catheter drainage** for 5 days.
   d. **Severe urethral disruption injuries**
      —are usually treated with suprapubic catheter placement, with **delayed repair** (3 months) of the urethral injury.
   e. **Primary repair of a urethral injury**
      —may be necessary with severe bladder neck lacerations or when pelvic vascular or rectal injuries are present.

4. **Complications** of these injuries include
   —urethral stricture.
   —incontinence.
   —impotence.

VI. Functional Disorders of the Genitourinary Tract

A. **Urinary incontinence**
   1. The **types of urinary incontinence**
      —are characterized in **Table 6-8.**
   2. **Evaluation**
      a. **Examination should include**
         —a full **neurologic assessment.**
         —**abdominal examination** for distended bladder.
         —**rectal examination** for tone and for assessment of the prostate.
      b. A **pelvic examination** with a full bladder assesses for
         —leakage with Valsalva maneuver.
         —cystocele.
         —rectocele.
      c. **Instillation of methylene blue**

Table 6-8. Types of Urinary Incontinence

Type of Incontinence	Mechanism	Findings	Treatment Options
Stress (anatomic)	Hypermobile urethra or loss of smooth sphincter function	Precipitated by coughing, sneezing, exercise, or position change	Kegel exercises, biofeedback, α_1-adrenergic agonists **Surgical:** urethral suspension, pubovaginal sling, periurethral collagen injection
Urge (detrusor instability)	Involuntary detrusor contractions **without** neurologic disorder	Sensation of urgency with frequency	Anticholinergics (oxybutynin); behavior modification; biofeedback; electrical stimulation **Surgical:** cystoplasty, urinary diversion
Neuropathic (detrusor hyperreflexia)	Involuntary detrusor **with** neurologic disorders	Urgency (when sensate), frequency, decreased bladder capacity; associated **neurologic conditions:** multiple sclerosis, spinal cord injury, stroke	Treat underlying neurologic condition; behavior modification, biofeedback, electrical stimulation **Surgical:** cystoplasty, urinary diversion
Overflow	Obstruction (BPH) leads to distension and leakage	Sensation of complete emptying and enlarged bladder	Correct obstructive process
Congenital	Sphincter mechanism bypassed	Continuous leakage and nocturnal enuresis	Surgical correction (e.g., ureteral ectopy, bladder exstrophy)
Fistulous	Postsurgical or inflammatory	Continuous leakage and nocturnal enuresis; IVP frequently diagnostic	Surgical correction: urethrovaginal, vesicovaginal, or ureterovaginal fistula
Traumatic	Pelvic fracture with anatomic injury, or neurologic injury, or both	Continuous leakage and nocturnal enuresis	Kegel exercises; biofeedback; periurethral collagen injections; artificial urinary sphincter

BPH = benign prostatic hyperplasia; IVP = intravenous pyelography.

—into the bladder and placement of a vaginal tampon can be used to assess for vesicovaginal fistula.

    d. **Urinalysis and culture**

        —should be performed to rule out infection or urolithiasis.

    e. **Uroflowmetry and postvoid residual**

—are useful initial tests to assess functional capacity.

f. Cystourethroscopy

—allows for **evaluation of bladder** mucosa for tumors.

—may identify ectopic ureters or vesicovaginal fistulae.

g. IVP, cystography, or retrograde pyelography

—are used to identify vesicovaginal or ureterovaginal fistulae, tumors, or ectopic ureters.

h. Urodynamic evaluation

—**assesses detrusor function and instability.**

—determines the etiology of incontinence (e.g., urethral hypermobility, intrinsic sphincter deficiency).

—characterizes the degree of pelvic prolapse in female patients.

3. Treatment options

—for each type of incontinence are outlined in **Table 6-8.**

B. Neurogenic bladder

1. The **bladder normally performs the dual functions** of low-pressure storage and voluntary micturition.

2. Control of these functions is exerted via the

—cerebral cortex.

—pons.

—sacral spinal cord and its nerve branches.

—These coordinate detrusor and external sphincter activity appropriately.

3. Diagnosis and classification

—are often made by urodynamic testing.

4. Disruption of normal anatomy

—can cause voiding dysfunction depending on the location of the lesion (**Table 6-9**).

Table 6-9. Neurogenic Bladder

Bladder Type	Causes(s)	Treatment(s)
Spastic Low capacity	Injury above T12	CIC + anticholinergics, Foley or condom catheter, sacral rhizotomy, urinary diversion, bladder augmentation + CIC
Normal capacity		Stimulated voiding, CIC + anticholinergics
Flaccid	Injury below T12 Neuropathy Trauma	Timed voiding Catheterization (clean or continuous)

CIC = clean intermittent catheterization.

5. Treatment

—**hinges on both** adequate urinary drainage (e.g., continuous or intermittent catheterization) and protection of the upper urinary tracts from damage caused by chronic increased pressure (over 40 cm H_2O intravesical) or infection.

C. Testicular torsion

1. Spontaneous torsion of the testicle

—can result in ischemia.

—is a surgical emergency.

2. Patients typically present during puberty with acute scrotal pain with elevation of the testicle.

3. The torted testis rotates internally (toward the penis).

4. If torsion is suspected clinically

—**emergent surgical exploration** is indicated to preserve testicular viability (less than 6 hours).

5. Doppler ultrasound

—may sometimes be used to demonstrate decreased testicular blood flow versus increased flow seen with epididymitis or orchitis.

6. Manual detorsion and orchiopexy

—are performed at the time of exploration.

—Nonviable testicles require removal.

D. Erectile dysfunction

1. Physiology of erection

a. Stimulation (e.g., audiovisual, tactile) is mediated through the pelvic plexus.

—Nerve terminals on corporal smooth muscle release **nitric oxide,** which causes relaxation of penile corporal smooth muscle.

b. Arterial dilation and simultaneous venous compression engorges the corporal bodies, conferring axial rigidity to the penis sufficient for penetration.

c. Detumescence and flaccidity is mediated by sympathetic tone.

2. Causes of erectile dysfunction

a. Vascular causes include

—inadequate arterial supply (e.g., atherosclerosis, trauma).

—excessive venous outflow (e.g., venous leak).

b. Neurogenic causes include

—diabetic neuropathy.

—CNS injury.

c. Endocrine causes include

—prolactinoma.

—hypogonadism.

—diabetes mellitus.

d. Iatrogenic causes include
—surgery (e.g., colectomy, prostatectomy).
—antihypertensive and antidepressant medications.

e. Psychogenic erectile dysfunction
—may be defined as insufficiency of erections when desired in the presence of a functional neurovascular system.
—may be due to increased sympathetic tone (anxiety), depression, or other complex CNS influences on erectile function.
—**Nocturnal erections are often but not always present.**

3. Diagnosis
—is often based on history and physical findings alone.

a. Document the presence or absence of
—other diseases.
—medications.
—nocturnal erections.
—neurologic findings (e.g., anal sphincter tone, perineal sensation).

b. Laboratory studies, while often unrewarding, may include
—luteinizing hormone.
—follicle-stimulating hormone (FSH).
—prolactin.
—serum testosterone.
—They are important to rule out a central nervous system cause of impotence.

c. Imaging with Doppler ultrasound
—after administration of vasoactive agents can assess penile arterial flow and detect venous leakage.

4. Treatment

a. An **oral agent [e.g., sildenafil (Viagra)]**
—may be tried empirically in the absence of contraindications, assuming CNS causes have been ruled out.
(1) Further work-up is often suspended if oral therapy is successful.
(2) Its use is **contraindicated** in patients using **nitrate preparations,** due to severe hypotension.

b. Intracorporal injection therapy
—requires direct injection of vasoactive agents (e.g., prostaglandin E_1) into the corpus cavernosum.

c. Penile prostheses
—are surgically inserted and confer mechanical rigidity to the penis.

d. Psychotherapy
—may play an important role, particularly in patients with psychogenic erectile dysfunction.

E. Priapism
—is a **prolonged** (longer than 4 hours), **often painful erection.**

—is characterized by rigidity of the corpora cavernosa but flaccidity of the glans penis.

1. **Etiologies**
   a. **Idiopathic causes** (most common)
   b. **Iatrogenic causes** (e.g., intracavernous injections for impotence)
   c. **Pathologic causes:**
      —sickle cell disease
      —hypercoagulable states
      —neurogenic causes
      —traumatic injuries

2. **Management** involves
   —treatment of any underlying disorder.

   —corporal aspiration and irrigation, followed by instillation of α-adrenergic agonist agents (e.g., phenylephrine).
   a. Embolization may be required in traumatic cases, or patients **refractory to more conservative treatment.**
   b. Surgical shunting procedures (e.g., cavernosum-spongiosum shunt) take advantage of separate drainage systems.

Review Test

Directions: Each of the numbered items or incomplete statements in this section is followed by answers or by completions of the statement. Select the ONE lettered answer or completion that is BEST in each case.

1. A 46-year-old man with a history of gout presents to the emergency room with severe flank pain. Work-up reveals uric acid crystals in the urine. Which of the following is an appropriate statement regarding the evaluation of this patient?

(A) This patient's urine pH is likely to be elevated
(B) These stones likely contain struvite in addition to uric acid
(C) A computed tomography (CT) scan will likely identify the location of these stones
(D) Gross or microscopic hematuria must be present
(E) This patient will likely give a history of high dietary calcium intake

2. A 32-year-old woman has a history of recurrent urinary tract infections (UTIs) over the past 3 years that generally resolve with oral antibiotic therapy. She now presents to the office with microscopic hematuria that persists despite clear urine. Before an intravenous pyelography (IVP), a plain abdominal radiograph is obtained which reveals a branched calcification in the region of the right kidney. The IVP confirms its presence in the collecting system. Which of the following most probably describes the major constituent of the stone?

(A) Calcium oxalate monohydrate
(B) Calcium oxalate dihydrate
(C) Magnesium ammonium phosphate
(D) Calcium phosphate
(E) Cystine

3. A 63-year-old, healthy man with severe benign prostatic hyperplasia (BPH) undergoes transurethral resection of the prostate (TURP) for recurrent urinary retention. The procedure lasts 55 minutes and there are no intraoperative complications. In the recovery room, he becomes confused and lethargic. The nurse calls you and tells she believes he is seizing. Which of the following tests is most appropriate in this setting?

(A) Chest radiograph
(B) Serum electrolytes
(C) Fingerstick glucose
(D) Electrocardiogram
(E) Electroencephalogram (EEG)

4. A 67-year-old smoker who is on no medications and has no known allergies presents to the office after a single episode of painless gross hematuria. Intravenous pyelography (IVP) reveals an irregular contour to the left kidney, but no other abnormalities in the kidneys, ureters, or bladder. Complete blood count and serum creatinine from 2 months earlier is normal. Flexible cystoscopy is unremarkable. Which of the following is the most appropriate next step in the evaluation of this patient?

(A) Computed tomography (CT)-guided needle biopsy of the mass
(B) T_2-weighted magnetic resonance imaging (MRI) of the abdomen
(C) CT scan of the abdomen with and without intravenous contrast
(D) Technetium bone scan
(E) Chest radiograph

5. A 66-year-old, otherwise healthy man presents for evaluation of erectile dysfunction. On rectal examination there is a discrete nodule on the right lobe of the prostate. His prostate-specific antigen (PSA) prior to examination is 0.8 ng/mL. Which of the following is the best next step in the management of this patient?

(A) Determine serum levels of luteinizing hormone and follicle-stimulating hormone
(B) Computed tomography (CT) scan of the head
(C) Prostatic biopsy
(D) Intracavernous injection therapy and recheck PSA in 6 months
(E) Sildenafil (Viagra) and recheck PSA in 6 months

6. A 52-year-old woman presents with complaints of sudden urge to void with subsequent urinary incontinence, and minor leakage with straining or coughing for the past 6 months. Which of the following treatment or evaluation measures would be contraindicated in this patient?

(A) Imipramine
(B) Behavioral feedback therapy
(C) Pubovaginal sling operation
(D) Urinalysis and urine culture
(E) Anticholinergic therapy

7. A 75-year-old, previously ambulatory man presents to the emergency department with sudden onset of lower extremity weakness. His family tells you he has a history of prostate cancer treated with radiation 6 years earlier. Spinal magnetic resonance imaging (MRI) reveals a mass with cord compression in the lumbar spine strongly suspicious for metastatic prostate cancer. Which of the following is most appropriate in the treatment of this patient?

(A) Immediate surgical decompression
(B) Leuprolide
(C) Flutamide
(D) Ketoconazole
(E) Diethylstilbestrol (DES)

8. A 57-year-old, diabetic, hypertensive man is referred with the complaint of erectile dysfunction. The patient takes multiple medications. He is inquiring about the use of sildenafil (Viagra) for the treatment of his erectile dysfunction. Among his medications listed below, which of the following is an *absolute* contraindication to the use of sildenafil?

(A) Doxazosin
(B) Isosorbide dinitrate
(C) Metformin
(D) Digoxin
(E) Procainamide

9. A 70-year-old, otherwise healthy man complains of worsening urinary hesitancy, nocturia, and diminished force of his urinary stream. He has had two culture-proven urinary tract infections (UTIs) in the past year. He currently takes an α_1-adrenergic blocker. His serum creatinine is 2.1 mg/dL and prostate-specific antigen (PSA) is normal. Which of the following is most appropriate in the management of this patient?

(A) Flutamide
(B) Increase doxazosin dose
(C) Transurethral resection of the prostate (TURP)
(D) Leuprolide injection therapy
(E) Finasteride

10. An 18-year-old man presents with a testicular mass palpable on examination and replacing 90% of the testis on ultrasound. Preoperative tests reveal serum α-fetoprotein (AFP) and β-human chorionic gonadotropin are normal. Computed tomography (CT) scan of the abdomen and chest radiograph are normal. Radical inguinal orchiectomy is performed. Histopathologic analysis reveals seminoma confined to the testis with early lymphovascular invasion. Which of the following best describes the appropriate management for this patient?

(A) Observation
(B) Prophylactic retroperitoneal lymph node dissection
(C) Prophylactic platinum-based chemotherapy
(D) Repeat serum tumor marker analysis CT scan and chest film in 3 months
(E) Retroperitoneal irradiation

11. You are present in the emergency room when a 35-year-old man arrives by helicopter after sustaining severe injuries in a motor vehicle accident. Preliminary radiographs reveal a severe pelvic fracture. The surgical team wishes to resuscitate the patient rapidly and wants a urinary catheter in place. Which of the following is the most appropriate management step in this patient?

(A) Condom catheter
(B) Attempt to gently pass a small catheter
(C) Wait for patient to void and then analyze urine
(D) Retrograde cystourethrogram
(E) Suprapubic catheter

12. A 15-year-old boy is complaining of 4 hours of right testicular pain. He denies trauma to the testis and previous episodes like this. His physical examination reveals an elevated, firm, and tender testicle, which seems to be in an unusual position. His temperature is 38° C. Urinalysis shows 2 to 3 red blood cells/high power field (hpf) and 4 white blood cells/hpf. Which of the following is the most appropriate next step?

(A) Nuclear scan for testicular blood flow
(B) Ultrasound of the testis
(C) Broad spectrum oral antibiotics for 7 days and follow-up
(D) Intravenous (IV) antibiotics
(E) Surgical exploration

13. A 67-year-old, male smoker presents after an episode of gross hematuria and left flank pain. He has never had a kidney stone. Non-contrast spiral computed tomography (CT) scan of the abdomen reveals an irregular mass in the left kidney but no stones. His serum creatinine is 0.9; hematocrit is 62%. What is the most likely explanation for the elevated hematocrit?

(A) Renal cyst
(B) Transitional cell carcinoma of the renal pelvis
(C) Dehydration
(D) Paraneoplastic syndrome
(E) Cigarette smoking

14. A 58-year-old, Egyptian man presents to your office with a referral for microscopic hematuria and urinary urgency. He has smoked one pack of cigarettes per day for 40 years. He takes hydrochlorothiazide for his blood pressure. Physical examination is unremarkable. Intravenous pyelography (IVP) is normal. On cystoscopy you notice an abnormal area of tissue near the bladder neck, and biopsy reveals squamous cell carcinoma. Which is the most likely causative factor in this diagnosis?

(A) _Echinococcus granulosus_
(B) Cigarette smoking
(C) _Dracunculus medinensis_
(D) _Schistosoma hematobium_
(E) Prostate carcinoma invading the bladder

15. You are evaluating a 50-year-old, hypertensive man with the complaint of intermittent left-sided flank pain for 2 months. On physical examination you notice that he has bilateral varicoceles and the patient states that he has had them as long as he can remember. In the supine position, the right-sided varicocele disappears, but the left-sided one persists. Which of the following choices best explains this finding?

(A) Drainage of the ipsilateral gonadal vein into the higher-pressure vena cava
(B) Drainage of the contralateral gonadal vein into the renal vein
(C) Cirrhosis with portal hypertension
(D) Vascular changes due to longstanding systemic hypertension
(E) Renal cell carcinoma (RCC) invading the left renal vein

Answers and Explanations

1-C. Essentially 100% of stones are detected on computed tomography (CT) scanning, regardless of composition. Indinavir, an antiretroviral, has been reported to cause radiolucent stones on CT scan. Uric acid stones form in an acid (low) pH, which favors precipitation of relatively insoluble uric acid. Most urinary stones are composed of calcium oxalate, not struvite (magnesium ammonium phosphate). Hematuria is often present to some degree, but is not considered necessary for diagnosis. Dietary calcium intake correlates poorly with stone formation.

2-C. In stone disease in the setting of recurrent urinary tract infections (UTIs), the diagnosis of struvite, or infection stones, should always be entertained. They result from urease-producing bacteria (e.g., _Proteus, Klebsiella_) which elevate urine pH via production of ammonia. This environment favors precipitation of magnesium ammonium phosphate crystals and staghorn stone formation. The other choices are less likely in this clinical scenario.

3-B. This question describes "transurethral resection (TUR) syndrome," which can complicate transurethral prostatectomy. Hypotonic irrigant solutions (e.g., water, glycine) can be introduced through venous channels in the prostate in sufficient quantity to cause dilutional hyponatremia and possibly hyperammonemia with use of glycine. Risk factors include prolonged operative time and excessive irrigant pressure. In this clinical setting, any of the other tests listed would be of limited benefit in confirming the diagnosis.

4-C. Computed tomography (CT) scan with and without contrast is the key diagnostic tool for parenchymal lesions. Solid renal masses should be considered malignant until proven otherwise. Needle biopsy does not alter the course of management, as negative or indeterminate biopsies are not reliable. Magnetic resonance imaging (MRI) of the abdomen may be necessary for a patient who cannot tolerate intravenous (IV) contrast or if renal vein involvement is suspected, but is generally not the first choice study in this scenario. Bone scan is not indicated at this point. Renal angiography may be helpful for very large tumors or abnormal anatomic situations, but is not a necessary part of the work-up of this patient with an otherwise normal intravenous pyelography (IVP).

5-C. A suspicious nodule on the prostate is an absolute indication for biopsy, regardless of prostate-specific antigen (PSA) level. Gonadotropin levels and computed tomography (CT) scan of the head may rule out rare but important pituitary causes (e.g., prolactinoma) of impotence, but are probably of little value in this scenario. Sildenafil (Viagra) or prostaglandin E_1 are reasonable therapies for this patient's erectile dysfunction, but the prostatic nodule requires immediate attention.

6-C. The pubovaginal sling operation is useful in the setting of stress incontinence, but can worsen or even create symptoms of urgency. Therefore it is contraindicated in the patient with significant urge symptoms. Imipramine, anticholinergics, and behavioral feedback therapy are all appropriate choices for treatment of urge incontinence. Urinalysis and urine culture are essential diagnostic tools in this setting.

7-D. Ketoconazole is a potent inhibitor of steroidogenesis and is useful for the rapid reduction of serum testosterone in emergent situations such as this. Adrenal suppression must be watched for as well. Luteinizing hormone-releasing hormone (LHRH) agonists may worsen the problem acutely due to the initial flare of testosterone levels. Flutamide will not affect testosterone levels and is a competitive inhibitor of androgen at the cellular level. Diethylstilbestrol (DES), a now rarely used synthetic estrogen, decreases testosterone by feedback inhibition over a period of days, but has thromboembolic risks associated with its use. Emergent radiotherapy would also be effective in this case.

8-B. Sildenafil (Viagra), a selective Type V phosphodiesterase inhibitor, can induce life-threatening hypotension in combination with nitrate-containing drugs. The other drugs listed are generally considered compatible with sildenafil use.

9-C. Transurethral resection of the prostate (TURP) is strongly indicated in this patient, who has had two urinary tract infections (UTIs) and azotemia resulting from his benign prostatic hyperplasia (BPH). Flutamide has no role in BPH management. A different α_1-antagonist is unlikely to be beneficial. Leuprolide or finasteride may ultimately improve the patient's symptoms, but this patient has failed medical therapy and requires more definitive intervention for his BPH.

10-E. This is an organ-confined seminoma, which is treated by orchiectomy and radiation therapy to the retroperitoneum. Chemotherapy and retroperitoneal lymph node dissection are not indicated given the stage and histology, respectively. Observation is inappropriate given the element of lymphovascular invasion. Most experts advocate the use of adjunctive radiation therapy (i.e., 3000 cGy) given its low morbidity and proven positive impact on survival.

11-D. Retrograde urethrogram should always be performed before attempting catheter insertion in this situation. There is a risk of worsening a partial injury in blind passage of a catheter. Suprapubic cystostomy should be performed in cases of confirmed urethral injury but does not precede performance of the urethrogram. Some experts prefer immediate realignment of the urethra. Placement of a condom catheter or waiting for the patient to void would not address the issue of a potential bladder or urethral injury in a timely manner.

12-E. Scrotal exploration is 100% sensitive and specific for torsion. In a high-suspicion case like this one, immediate exploration is warranted. Additional tests may delay definitive treatment. Doppler ultrasound may be helpful in equivocal cases to demonstrate intratesticular blood flow.

13-D. This patient has erythrocytosis, which is a known syndrome associated with renal cell carcinoma (RCC), and an irregular mass is noted on this patient's noncontrast computed tomography (CT) scan for stones. Smoking and dehydration can also cause a mild elevation of hematocrit, but not usually to this degree. Transitional cell carcinoma of the renal pelvis is not associated with erythrocytosis.

14-D. Squamous cell carcinoma is an unusual cancer in the bladder, and it is often associated with schistosomiasis (bilharziasis), particularly in a patient fitting this description. Chronic irritation (e.g., foreign bodies) is causative. Smoking is associated with transitional cell carcinoma.

15-E. Varicoceles that do not disappear in the supine position raise the suspicion of retroperitoneal malignancy until proven otherwise. Varicoceles form more commonly on the left side, as the gonadal vein empties into the higher pressure renal vein, which contributes to retrograde flow and testicular damage. Long-standing hypertension has no known correlation with varicocele; neither does cirrhosis with portal hypertension because varicocele involves the systemic venous circulation, not the portal system.

7

Neurosurgery

Jeffrey J. Laurent, Tord D. Alden,
John A. Jane, Jr., Jonas M. Sheehan

I. Trauma

A. General

1. A **computed tomography (CT) scan should be performed**
   —if there is a history of loss of consciousness.
   —if the **Glascow Coma Score (GCS) is less than 15 (Table 7-1).**

2. **Management of head injury** includes
   —volume resuscitation, avoiding hypotension.
   —rapid diagnostic evaluation.
   —prophylactic antiseizure medication if there is an intracranial lesion.
   —intracranial pressure (ICP) monitoring.

3. **Elevated ICP**
   a. **Signs** include
      —bradycardia (early).
      —respiratory irregularity (late).
      —hypertension (late) (**Cushing's triad**).
   b. **A sixth nerve palsy**
      —can be indicative of increased ICP.
   c. **ICP**
      —correlates with outcome.
      —is a component of cerebral perfusion pressure (CPP):

      CPP = mean arterial pressure (MAP) − ICP.

   d. **ICP monitoring should be used**
      —if increased ICP is suspected.

Table 7-1. Glasgow Coma Scale

Points	Best Eye Response	Best Verbal Response	Best Motor Response
6	—	—	Obeys commands
5	—	Oriented	Localizes to pain
4	Open spontaneously	Confused	Withdraws from pain
3	Open to voice	Inappropriate	Flexion (decorticate)
2	Open to pain	Incomprehensible sounds	Extension (decerebrate)
1	None	None	None

—if neurologic examination is not possible (e.g., unconscious patient, pharmacological sedation).

e. **Treatment measures** include
—elevating the head of the bed.
—sedation/pharmacological paralysis.
—hyperventilation (for acute increase in ICP, not chronic).
—osmotic diuretics (mannitol).
—barbiturate coma.
—decompressive craniectomy (**Kjellberg procedure**).

B. **Skull fractures**

1. **Linear fractures**

—generally require no treatment.

2. **Depressed fractures**
a. **Depressed fractures should be elevated** if there
—is **more than 8–10 mm depression.**
—is underlying brain injury.
—are open fractures.
—is frontal sinus violation, or a cerebrospinal fluid (CSF) leak.
b. These fractures must be closely monitored for postoperative infection.

3. **Temporal fractures**

—may result in injury to cranial nerve (CN) VII and VIII.

4. **Basilar fractures**
a. **Characteristics** of basilar fractures include
—**CSF otorrhea or rhinorrhea.**
—**hemotympanum.**
—**Battle's sign** (postauricular ecchymoses).
—periorbital ecchymoses (**"raccoon eyes"**).
—injury to CN I, VII, or VIII.
b. **Many basilar skull fractures** do not require treatment.

C. **Epidural hematoma (Figure 7.1)**

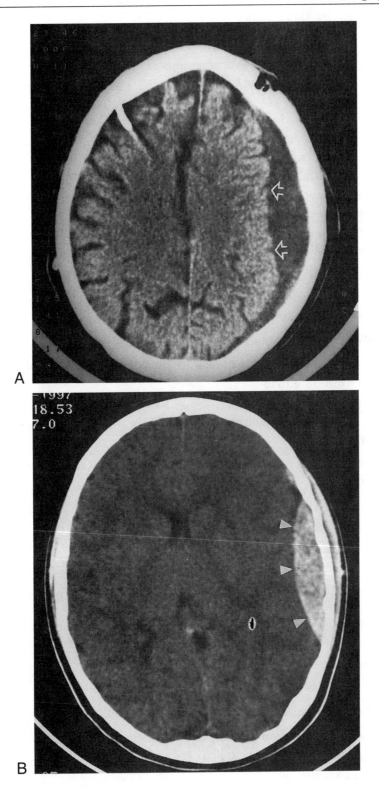

Figure 7.1. Computed tomography (CT) scan of an acute subdural and epidural hematoma. (*A*) CT scan **with intravenous (IV) contrast** showing a subacute subdural hematoma. (*B*) CT scan **without IV contrast** showing an acute epidural hematoma. (Reprinted with permission from Daffner RH: *Clinical Radiology: The Essentials,* 2nd ed. Baltimore, Williams & Wilkins, 1999, p 19 and 513.)

—is defined as blood above the dura.

1. **The classic scenario (10%–25%) includes, in order,**
   a. post-traumatic loss of consciousness.
   b. a **"lucid interval."**
   c. and later
      —decreased level of consciousness.
      —vomiting.
      —restlessness.
      —death **(20%–40%).**

2. **Eight-five percent of cases are caused by** bleeding from the **middle meningeal artery.**

3. **CT scan will show** a **biconvex** (lenticular—like a lens) area of high density abutting the skull without crossing suture lines.

4. **Treatment** includes
   —surgical evacuation.
   —cautery of bleeding vessels.

D. **Subdural hematoma** (see Figure 7.1)

—is defined as blood under the dura but above the arachnoid layer.

1. **A common cause**
   —involves tearing of a surface or **bridging vessel** (usually veins) from acceleration/deceleration of brain.

2. **Mortality**
   —is reported at 50%–90% and is generally related to brain injury.

3. **CT scan**
   —shows a high-density **crescent-shaped** mass adjacent to the skull (see Figure 7-1).

4. **Treatment**
   —is emergent evacuation in the operating room.

5. **Chronic subdural hematomas usually occur** in the elderly, sometimes weeks to months after a trivial incident.
   —Surgical evacuation is performed for symptomatic or large lesions (larger than 1 cm).

E. **Traumatic subarachnoid hemorrhage (SAH)**

—is defined as blood below the arachnoid layer and above the pia.

—**Management** is with prophylactic anticonvulsants.

F. **Traumatic intraventricular hemorrhage (IVH)**

—may cause hydrocephalus, which requires ventricular drainage (ventriculostomy).

G. **Cerebral contusions**

—are caused by head trauma with the brain forced against the skull.

1. **On CT they appear as** small areas of hemorrhage.
2. These **contusions are classified** as **coup** and **contrecoup** injuries.
   a. **Coup:** injury to the brain at the point of impact
   b. **Contrecoup:** blows to the head forcing the brain against the skull opposite to the direct blow
3. **Treatment** involves

   —anticonvulsant prophylaxis.

   —diligent monitoring.

H. Diffuse axonal injury

—appears as small areas of hemorrhage deep in the white matter.

1. **Treatment** involves anticonvulsant prophylaxis.
2. The **prognosis** for this injury is very poor.

I. Spinal cord injuries

—are classified as complete or incomplete.

1. **Complete lesions**

   —present with no function below the level of injury.

2. **Incomplete lesions**

   —are associated with some retained function (either motor or sensory) below the level of injury.
   a. **Preservation of proprioception**

      —of the lower extremities may be present.
   b. **"Sacral sparing"** is indicated by

      —voluntary **anal sphincter** contraction.

      —perianal sensation.

      —toe flexion.

3. **Clinical syndromes**

   —seen with spinal cord injury are outlined in **Table 7-2.**

4. **Immobilization is key**

   —to reduce the risk of further injury.

5. **Treatment essential for these injuries**
   a. **Adequate resuscitation**

      —with systolic blood pressure (SBP) over 90 mm Hg.
   b. **Early administration of methylprednisolone**

      —for 24 hours if given within 0–3 hours of injury.

      —for 48 hours if initiated 3–8 hours after injury.

6. **Patient must remain in a cervical collar**

   —until it is confirmed that there is no evidence of a C-spine injury (through T1).
   a. **No abnormalities** on anteroposterior (AP), lateral, or odontoid films in a coherent patient

Table 7-2. Clinical Syndromes Seen in Spinal Cord Injury

Syndrome	Associated Injury	Signs and Symptoms	Prognosis
Brown-Séquard syndrome	**Cord hemisection,** frequently due to penetrating trauma	**Ipsilateral paralysis and proprioception loss;** contralateral loss of pain and temperature sensation below the injury	Up to 90% of patients with this injury will recover function sufficient to ambulate
Anterior spinal syndrome	Infarction of the area of the cord supplied by the **anterior spinal artery;** cause may be vascular or compressive	Bilateral paralysis with loss of pain and temperature but **preservation of dorsal column function** (e.g., proprioception)	Approximately 10% will recover to ambulate independently
Central cord syndrome	Frequently follows **hyperextension injury** in patients with preexisting bony hypertrophy and canal stenosis	**Motor weakness** of the upper extremities with less effect on the lower extremities	About 50% will recover to ambulate independently

   b. **No neck pain** or neurologic deficits on flexion/extension/lateral movement

J. **Spinal fractures**

   1. **Cervical spine**

      a. A **Jefferson fracture**

         —is through the **arch of C1.**

         —is commonly caused by axial compression.

      b. A **Hangman's fracture**

         —is through the **pars interarticularis of C2.**

      c. **Odontoid fractures are divided into three types**

         (1) **I:** through tip of dens

         (2) **II:** through neck (base) of dens

         (3) **III:** through the body of C2 **(Figure 7.2)**

      d. **Clay shoveler's fracture**

         —involve the spinous processes **(usually C7).**

      e. **Unilateral or bilateral jumped facets**

         —usually result from hyperflexion injury with rotation and associated ligamentous disruption.

   2. **Thoracolumbar**

      a. **The 3 columns of the thoracolumbar spine include (Figure 7.3)**

         (1) **Anterior:** anterior longitudinal ligament and anterior half of vertebral body.

         (2) **Middle:** posterior half of vertebral body and posterior longitudinal ligament.

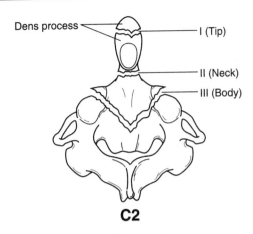

Figure 7.2. Three types of odontoid fractures. (Adapted with permission from Blackbourne L: *Advanced Surgical Recall.* Baltimore, Williams & Wilkins, 1998, p 1211.)

    (3) Posterior: facet joints, lamina, spinous processes, interspinous ligament.

  b. If more than 1 column is disrupted, an injury is considered **unstable.**

  c. Compression fractures
    —usually involve the anterior column only (**stable** injury).

  d. Burst fractures
    —are considered unstable fractures (i.e., 2 columns are disrupted).
    —usually require spinal fusion using instrumentation.

  e. CT scans
    —can complement plain radiographs in the evaluation of spinal injuries.

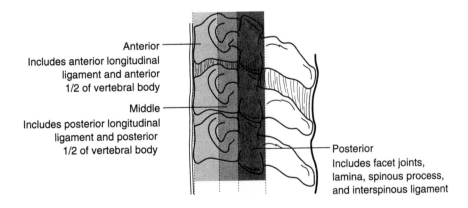

Figure 7.3. The three columns of the thoracolumbar spine. **Anterior column** includes an anterior longitudinal ligament and anterior half of the vertebral body. **Middle column** includes a posterior longitudinal ligament and posterior half of the vertebral body. **Posterior column** includes facet joints, lamina, spinous process, and interspinous ligament. (Adapted with permission from Blackbourne L: *Advanced Surgical Recall.* Baltimore, Williams & Wilkins, 1998, p 1210.)

3. **Indications for emergent magnetic resonance imaging** (MRI) include

—a worsening neurologic deficit.

—suspected soft tissue injury in the absence of bony injury.

—a fracture level inconsistent with injury level.

4. **Indications for emergent decompressive surgery** include

—fracture or dislocation not reducible by distraction (e.g., jumped facet).

—acute anterior cord syndrome.

—open fracture.

—penetrating trauma.

—radiographic demonstration of soft tissue compression of the cord.

—progressive neurologic deterioration.

II. Adult and Pediatric Tumors of the Brain and Spinal Cord (Table 7-3)

A. **General**

1. **The most common primary brain tumors are gliomas** (e.g., astrocytomas, oligodendrogliomas, ependymomas).

—They **account for 50%** of all lesions.

2. **Two thirds of**

—**adult** brain tumors are **supratentorial.**

—**pediatric** tumors are **infratentorial.**

3. **The most common presenting symptoms of brain tumors** are

—headache (typically worse in the morning).

—progressive neurologic deficits.

—seizures.

a. The **headache** is often temporarily relieved by vomiting.

b. Other signs and symptoms vary according to tumor location (**Table 7-4**).

4. **Radiologic studies**

—are essential to the diagnosis of brain tumors.

a. **A ring enhancing lesion may represent**

—metastatic carcinoma.

—abscess.

—glioblastoma multiforme.

—lymphoma.

b. **Cystic tumors include**

—pilocytic astrocytomas.

—hemangioblastoma.

—craniopharyngiomas.

Table 7-3. Incidence of the Most Common Tumors of the Brain

Intra-axial Brain Tumors

Glioma	50%
Glioblastoma multiforme	50%
Low-grade astrocytoma	30%
Anaplastic astrocytoma	10%
Ependymoma	5%
Oligodendroglioma	5%
Metastases	20%
Meningioma	15%
Neuroma	5%
Medulloblastoma	5%
Pituitary adenomas	3%
Craniopharyngioma	2%

Infratentorial Pediatric Brain Tumors

Medulloblastomas	30%
Cerebellar astrocytoma	30%
Ependymoma	20%
Brainstem glioma	10%
Miscellaneous	10%
Choroid plexus papilloma	
Hemangioblastoma	
Epidermoid/dermoid	
Chordoma	

    c. **Areas of calcification may be present** in
        —oligodendrogliomas.
        —ependymomas.
        —meningiomas.
        —craniopharyngiomas.

  B. Astrocytoma

    1. **Astrocytomas** may be **diffuse** or **circumscribed.**

      a. **Circumscribed lesions**
        —have a favorable prognosis (common in children).

      b. **Diffuse lesions**
        —are the most common type (75%).
        —have a poor prognosis (e.g., glioblastoma multiforme).
        —The peak age is 35–40.

Table 7-4. Presenting Signs and Symptoms of Brain Tumors by Location

Tumor Location	Presenting Signs and Symptoms
Infratentorial	Signs and symptoms of increased ICP: headache, nausea, vomiting, papilledema, gait disturbance, vertigo, diplopia
Supratentorial	Signs and symptoms of increased ICP plus unilateral focal motor deficits of entire limbs, seizures, mental status changes, personality changes (frontal lobes)
Cerebellar hemispheres	Signs and symptoms of increased ICP plus ataxia of the extremities, dysmetria, and intention tremor
Cerebellar vermis	Signs and symptoms of increased ICP plus broad-based gait, truncal ataxia, and titubation
Brainstem	Unilateral or bilateral 8th nerve palsies and/or 6th nerve palsies; multiple ipsilateral cranial nerve deficits with contralateral long tract signs, and vertical or rotary nystagmus; signs and symptoms of increased ICP occur late in the course

ICP = intracranial pressure.

2. **Two-year mortality with glioblastoma multiforme** is 90% despite treatment.
   a. These **tumors can cross** the corpus callosum, giving a butterfly appearance on CT.
   b. **Treatment** may involve
      —surgical debulking for symptomatic relief.
      —radiation with chemotherapy.
3. **Cerebellar astrocytomas**
   —occur most frequently between 3–20 years of age.
   a. **Treatment** involves surgical resection.
   b. **Malignant cerebellar astrocytomas** have a 29% 10-year survival.

C. **Brainstem gliomas**

—are generally malignant.

—affect children younger than 10 years old.

1. These tumors can be either **focal** or **diffuse.**
2. **Treatment** includes radiation therapy combined with steroids.
3. Most patients with malignant brainstem gliomas die within 1 year.

D. **Oligodendrogliomas**

—have a peak incidence between 35–45 years of age.

1. Patients with these tumors classically have a **long history of seizures.**
2. These lesions occur most commonly in the frontal lobe and are often **calcified.**
3. The prognosis varies, but overall 5-year survival is 40%.

E. Ependymomas

—can occur between ages 3–50 years, with a peak age of 10–15 years.

1. In **children,** most lesions are **intracranial.**

—The posterior fossa and spinal cord are the most common sites in adults.

2. Overall 5-year survival is 70%.

F. Meningiomas

—represent 15%–20% of all intracranial tumors.

1. Meningiomas

—occur most commonly between 40–50 years of age and are **twice as common in women** than men.

—**arise** from **arachnoid** cells, not the dura mater.

2. Symptoms

—are location dependent, but **proptosis** and **seizures** are common.

3. Histology

—**reveals psammoma bodies** and whorl formation.

—The criterion for malignancy is brain invasion.

4. Plain skull films

—may show bony destruction or hyperostosis.

—Meningiomas produce osteoblastic growth factors that cause bony overgrowth.

5. Treatment

—for accessible symptomatic lesions is by **surgical excision.**

6. Survival

—Meningiomas have a 91% 5-year survival, although some may recur.

G. Craniopharyngiomas

—are pediatric tumors, occurring between ages 3–10 years.

1. These tumors most frequently present with

—**endocrine abnormalities.**

—headache.

—visual field deficits.

—hydrocephalus.

2. Treatment

—is by surgical resection.

—Diabetes insipidus is a common postoperative complication.

3. Five-year survival

—is 55%–85%, with a 40% postoperative recurrence rate.

H. Medulloblastomas

—are the **most common primary brain tumors** in **children.**

1. These tumors arise from the cerebellum.

2. Because of their location, medulloblastomas often cause obstructive hydrocephalus associated with **headache, nausea or vomiting, and ataxia.**

3. These tumors have a tendency for **subarachnoid spread.**

4. **Treatment**

   —is with surgical debulking and radiation therapy.

   —These are highly radiosensitive tumors.

5. **Five-year survival** is 56%.

I. **Vestibular schwannomas**

1. Vestibular schwannomas **(acoustic neuromas)** arise from the superior vestibular portion of CN VIII.

   a. These tumors most commonly occur in middle-aged women.

   b. Bilateral tumors are diagnostic of neurofibromatosis type II (see VIII D).

2. **Patients typically present** with hearing loss, tinnitus, and dysequilibrium.

   —This is followed by facial numbness, ataxia, facial weakness and taste disturbance.

3. **Treatment**

   —is with surgical excision.

J. **Cerebral metastases**

—are the **most common tumors affecting the brain.**

1. **In adults, metastatic lesions** most commonly originate from tumors of the

   —lung (oat-cell carcinoma most common).

   —breast.

   —renal cell.

   —melanoma.

   —gastrointestinal tract.

2. The **most common sources of metastases in children** are

   —neuroblastoma.

   —rhabdomyosarcoma.

   —Wilms' tumor.

3. **A thorough search for the primary lesion is essential** for choosing specific **treatment** measures based on the characteristic of the primary tumor.

4. **Treatment for multiple metastases** includes both

   —medical treatment (e.g., anticonvulsants, dexamethasone, H_2 blockers).

   —radiation.

—**Symptomatic solitary lesions should be excised if the lesion is accessible.**

K. **Tumors of the spine and spinal cord**

—including extradural and intradural tumors are listed in **Table 7-5.**

1. Of **central nervous system (CNS) tumors** roughly 15% are intraspinal.

2. **Common presenting symptoms** of spinal tumors include

—pain.

—weakness.

—sensory disturbances.

—genitourinary/sphincter disturbances.

3. **Tumors of the conus medullaris or cauda equina**

—can present with characteristic constellations of symptoms.

a. **Conus medullaris**

(1) Onset is sudden.

(2) Symptoms are symmetric: the conus is the compact end of the cord; a lesion is going to affect the entire conus and cause bilateral symptoms.

(3) Pain and motor loss are not prominent, but sphincter disturbance is and occurs early.

Table 7-5. Tumors of the Spine and Spinal Cord

Extradural Tumors

Vertebral hemangioma
Chordoma
Neurofibroma
Osteoblastoma
Osteoid osteoma
Aneurysmal bone cysts

Metastatic Extradural Tumors

Prostate (osteoblastic)
Breast
Lung
Multiple myeloma
Lymphoma

Intradural Extramedullary Tumors

Meningioma
Neurofibroma

Intradural Intramedullary Tumors

Ependymomas
Astrocytomas
Others
    Teratoma
    Dermoid
    Epidermoid
    Malignant glioblastoma
    Hemangioblastoma

b. Cauda equina

(1) Onset is gradual.

(2) Symptoms are asymmetric: the cauda carries the nerve roots of the lower cord and is more spread out than the conus; a lesion here would have to involve nearly the entire canal to cause bilateral symptoms.

(3) Pain and motor loss are prominent and autonomic symptoms do not occur until late.

4. Diagnosis is based on

—clinical presentation.

—plain films.

—CT myelogram.

—MRI.

—angiographic findings.

5. Unlike infectious lesions, **tumors generally do not cross the intervertebral disk,** as demonstrated on CT or MRI.

6. Treatment

a. Radiation therapy and steroids are the first line of treatment.

b. Solitary lesions diagnosed early may be amenable to surgical resection.

III. Neuroendocrine

A. Pituitary adenomas

—arise from the anterior lobe of the pituitary.

1. The **age range** for these tumors is approximately 20–60 years.

2. Pituitary adenomas are sometimes **associated** with **multiple endocrine neoplasia (MEN) I** (see *BRS General Surgery,* Chapter 20 VI B).

3. Tumors present either because of endocrine dysfunction or mass effect with visual symptoms.

4. Some patients present with pituitary apoplexy, which is hemorrhage into the tumor requiring emergent surgery to preserve vision and pituitary function.

5. The **most common functional adenomas secrete**

—adrenocorticotropic hormone (ACTH).

—prolactin.

—growth hormone (GH).

6. Laboratory studies should include

—morning cortisol.

—thyroxine (T_4).

—thyroid stimulating hormone (TSH).

—follicle-stimulating hormone (FSH).

—luteinizing hormone (LH).

—estradiol or testosterone.

—GH.

—insulin-like growth factor (IGF)-1.

—prolactin.

—fasting glucose.

B. Cushing's syndrome

—is the general term for the constellation of symptoms caused by hyper-cortisolism (see *BRS General Surgery,* Chapter 20 III A).

1. Cushing's disease

—consists of an elevated ACTH caused by a pituitary adenoma.

2. Characteristic signs, symptoms, and diagnostic techniques

—of Cushing's disease are similar to those of Cushing's syndrome (see *BRS General Surgery,* Chapter 20 III A 2).

3. Measurement of ACTH

—in the inferior petrosal sinuses with comparisons to peripheral blood levels can sometimes be used to **localize the tumor,** either to the pituitary or to one side of the pituitary.

4. Treatment

—of Cushing's disease involves surgical resection of the adenoma.

C. Prolactinomas

1. Excess prolactin secretion

—can be caused by prolactinomas or by conditions interfering with the inhibitory action of dopamine on prolactin secretion.

a. Disruption of the pituitary stalk may lead to hyperprolactinemia.

b. Dopamine-blocking drugs (e.g., phenothiazines, cimetidine) may also cause hyperprolactinemia.

2. Symptoms

—of excess prolactin include infertility and impotence in men, and amenorrhea or galactorrhea in women.

3. Medical treatment

—with **bromocriptine, a dopamine agonist,** is warranted with prolactin levels over 500.

4. Surgery

—is indicated if medical treatment fails.

D. Acromegaly

—is caused by oversecretion of GH.

1. In children, excess GH may cause gigantism because the epiphyseal plates have not fused.

2. **Signs and symptoms of increased GH secretion** include

—frontal bogging, prognathic jaw, wide-spaced teeth.

—increase in hat, shoe, or ring size.

—thickened skin.

—hypertension and cardiomyopathy.

—carpal tunnel syndrome.

—headache.

—skin tags.

—excessive perspiration.

—sleep apnea.

—joint pain.

—deepened voice.

3. **Elevated fasting GH levels (over 10 ng/mL)**

—is suggestive of acromegaly.

—Elevated **somatomedin-C (IGF-1)** may also indicate acromegaly and is the most reliable method for biochemical diagnosis.

a. A glucose tolerance test is the gold standard to confirm the diagnosis in this setting.

b. Many GH-secreting adenomas also secrete prolactin.

4. The **best initial treatment**

—for acromegaly is **transsphenoidal resection.**

5. If **surgery fails or is incomplete**

—medical treatment with **octreotide** can be attempted.

E. **Nonfunctioning pituitary adenomas**

1. **Most pituitary tumors** presenting with mass effect are nonfunctional.

—Presentation is characteristic of the structure affected.

a. **Optic chiasm:** bitemporal hemianopsia

b. **Pituitary hypofunction** (e.g., hypothyroidism, diabetes insipidus)

c. **Cavernous sinus:** dysfunction of CN III, IV, V_1, V_2, VI

2. **Treatment**

—is by transsphenoidal resection of the lesion.

a. Patients should receive perioperative **hydrocortisone** to prevent hypocortisolemia after resection.

b. **Postoperative diabetes insipidus** also can be treated with fluids and DDAVP (an arginine vasopressin).

IV. Vascular Neurosurgery

A. **Nontraumatic subarachnoid hemorrhage (SAH)**

1. **Nontraumatic SAH is usually due to** rupture of a cerebral aneurysm (80%) or arteriovenous malformation (AVM) (5%).

—The cause is unknown in 15%.

2. **Signs and symptoms** of SAH include

—headache: classically described as **"worst headache of my life."**

—nuchal rigidity.

—nausea and vomiting.

—photophobia.

—neurologic deficits.

3. **Diagnosis**

a. A **CT scan is diagnostic**

—in most cases if performed within the first 48 hours.

b. **Xanthochromic CSF**

—is seen in 90% of patients within 12 hours of rupture.

c. **Cerebral angiography**

—helps to localize the bleeding site.

B. **Cerebral aneurysm**

1. **Most aneurysms (85%) are located** in the **anterior** (i.e., carotid) **circulation.**

—Twenty to 30% have multiple aneurysms.

2. The **etiology of cerebral aneurysms** may include

—congenital predisposition.

—connective tissue disease.

—embolic (e.g., as in atrial myxoma).

—infectious (mycotic aneurysms).

3. **Aneurysms frequently present** with rupture; however, they can also present with **mass effect, seizures,** and **infarcts** due to distal embolization.

4. **Untreated ruptured aneurysms**

—have a **significant rebleeding rate** (30% within 14 days, 50% within 6 months) with a 50%–60% mortality.

5. **Treatment**

—involves **surgical clipping of the aneurysm.**

—Endovascular therapies such as coiling and stenting are also evolving for aneurysm obliteration in surgically inaccessible lesions.

6. **Complications** include

—hydrocephalus.

—stroke.

—**arterial vasospasm.**

7. **Vasospasm may occur** 3–14 days after rupture, contributing to a 12% mortality rate.

C. **Arteriovenous malformations (AVMs)**

—are the **most common cause of SAH in children.**

1. The **most common symptoms and signs** include

   —headache.

   —epilepsy.

   —a progressive neurologic deficit.

2. **CT and MRI are reliable diagnostic studies.**

   —**Angiography,** however, provides the most precise preoperative map of the feeding and draining vessels.

3. **Hemorrhage from AVMs** rarely causes significant vasospasm.

4. If technically feasible, **symptomatic AVMs** should be **surgically excised.**

5. The **general risk of rupture** is about 2%–4% per year for AVMs.

   a. **Smaller AVMs bleed more frequently than larger ones.**

   b. The mortality is 10% with each rupture.

   c. The initial rebleeding rate is 10%–20%, returning to 2%–4% per year after 6 months.

6. **Owing to the risk of rupture,** asymptomatic AVMs should also be excised.

D. **Cerebrovascular occlusive disease and stroke**

   —(see Chapter 1 IV).

V. Degenerative Spine and Disc Disease

A. **Cervical disc disease**

1. Cervical discs affect the **nerve root** exiting **at the level** of the disc (i.e., nucleus pulposis compresses the C6 nerve root exiting between C5 and C6).

2. **Signs of cervical disc herniation (Table 7-6).**

   a. **Pain**

      —is worsened by neck extension and relieved by elevating the arm and holding it behind the head.

   b. **Spurling's sign**

      —refers to radicular pain reproduced by tilting or turning the head toward the side of pain and adding axial pressure.

3. A **large central cervical disk**

   —can produce signs and symptoms of spinal cord compression (e.g., spasticity, hyperreflexia).

4. **Surgery** can be performed

   —from the **back** (cervical laminectomy) if the disk is lateral or paracentral.

   —from the **front** (anterior cervical diskectomy and fusion) if the herniated disc is more centrally located.

B. **Cervical stenosis**

Table 7-6. Spinal Disc Disease

Disc Level	Presenting Signs and Symptoms
Cervical discs	
C4–C5 (1%)	C5 root affected Weakness of deltoid Pain over shoulder
C5–C6 (20%)	C6 root affected **Decreased biceps reflex** Weak forearm flexion Pain in upper arm, thumb, and forearm
C6–C7 (67%)	C7 root compressed **Diminished triceps reflex** Weakness of forearm extension Pain in index and middle fingers
C7–T1 (12%)	C8 root compressed Weakness of intrinsic hand muscles Pain in fourth and fifth fingers
Lumbar discs	
L3–L4 (5%)	Compress the L4 nerve root **Decreased patellar reflex** **Quadriceps weakness** **Decreased sensation over the medial malleolus** Pain in anterior thigh
L4–L5 (45%)	L5 nerve root compressed **Weakness of extensor hallucis longus and tibialis anterior (foot drop)** **Decreased sensation over big toe web space** Pain in lateral leg
L5–S1 (50%)	Compresses S1 nerve root **Diminished ankle jerk** **Weakness in plantar flexion of the foot** **Decreased sensation of lateral foot** Pain in posterior lower extremity

1. This **condition usually presents** with signs and symptoms of myelopathy with cord compression (upper motor neuron signs) or nerve root compression.

2. **MRI or CT myelography**

   —may reveal canal stenosis with cord compression.

3. **Surgical decompression**

   —is indicated if myelopathy is present.

C. **Lumbar disc herniation** (see Table 7-6)

   —often occurs in middle to older-aged individuals.

1. The **herniated nucleus pulposus** impinges on the nerve exiting at **the level below the disc** (L4–L5 disc compresses the L5 root exiting between L5–S1).

2. The most common **presenting symptom** is **back pain.**

—Other common features vary according to the level involved (see table 7-6).

a. Sciatica

—is defined as pain in a radicular pattern along the distribution of any of the lumbosacral nerve roots.

b. A positive straight leg raise test

—occurs when patients experience **pain in a radicular pattern** upon raising each leg against resistance while in the supine position.

3. An **MRI** can be diagnostic, but **CT myelography** remains the gold standard.

4. Most **patients respond** to **conservative therapy** [i.e., nonsteroidal anti-inflammatory drugs (NSAIDS), bed rest, physical therapy].

5. **Disc fragments that have herniated** through the annulus fibrosis often require **surgical removal.**

a. Eighty-five percent of patients with lumbar disc herniation will improve without surgery.

b. Thus, most surgeons advocate waiting 5–8 weeks from the onset of symptoms before performing surgery.

6. **Emergent surgery**

—is indicated for patients with **cauda equina syndrome or progressive motor deficits** (see II K 3 b).

—Compression of the cauda equina may cause bowel and bladder dysfunction as well as perianal anesthesia.

D. Lumbar stenosis

1. Spinal stenosis

—most commonly results from degenerative changes in the lumbar spine seen in the elderly.

2. Lumbar stenosis

—often presents as **neurogenic claudication.**

a. This is **characterized by** leg discomfort precipitated by prolonged standing or walking, relieved by sitting or lying down.

b. **Claudication** secondary to peripheral vascular disease must be ruled out.

3. MRI or CT myelogram

—may reveal stenosis of the canal and neural foramina.

4. Initial treatment

—includes NSAIDS and physical therapy.

—Surgical decompression is reserved for refractory signs and symptoms.

E. Spondylolysis and spondylolisthesis

1. Spondylolysis

—is a bony defect of the neural arch (pars interarticularis).

—may be congenital or traumatic.

—is often seen in adolescent gymnasts or football linemen owing to repetitive hyperextension stress on the lumbar spine.

2. **Spondylolisthesis**

—is **forward subluxation** or slip of **one vertebral body over the other.**

—most commonly occurs in the lower lumbar spine.

a. Spondylolisthesis typically presents with low back pain with or without radicular pain.

—This is **the most common cause of lumbar pain in adolescents.**

b. Lateral and oblique films of the spine will show subluxation or a pars defect.

c. **Treatment**

—depends on the degree of subluxation and symptoms.

(1) **Conservative treatment** involves activity modification, rest, and bracing.

(2) **Surgical fusion** of the vertebral bodies stabilizes the bodies and prevents further subluxation.

(3) **Decompression of the nerve roots** may be necessary if the patient suffers from persistent radicular symptoms.

VI. Pediatric Neurosurgery

A. **Subependymal hemorrhage**

—is seen in premature infants, usually less than 32 weeks' gestation.

—is secondary to rupture of fragile capillaries in the subependymal **germinal matrix.**

1. Eighty percent will proceed to intraventricular hemorrhage.

2. **Risk factors** include

—volume expansion.

—hypercapnia.

—cyanotic heart disease.

—extracorporeal membrane oxygenation (ECMO).

3. **Presenting symptoms** include

—neurologic deterioration.

—bulging fontanelles.

—a drop in blood pressure and hematocrit.

4. **Treatment**

—involves control of associated hydrocephalus with ventricular drainage by daily lumbar puncture or with placement of a ventricular catheter.

—A ventriculoperitoneal shunt may be necessary for long-term hydrocephalus.

B. **Hydrocephalus**

—is an abnormal increase in CSF volume associated with dilation of all or part of the ventricular system.

1. **Hydrocephalus is classified** as communicating or noncommunicating.
   a. **Communicating hydrocephalus**
      (1) CSF exits the brain without difficulty, but **outflow is blocked** at the level of the arachnoid granulations.
      (2) This may be caused by infection or hemorrhage leading to scarring of the arachnoid granulations.
   b. **Noncommunicating hydrocephalus**
      (1) Flow of CSF is obstructed at some point prior to its exit from the brain via the foramina of Magendie (midline) and Luschka (lateral).
      (2) Causes include stenosis of the cerebral aqueduct and masses that compress the ventricular system.
      (3) This occurs postoperatively in 20% of pediatric patients.
2. **Shunting of CSF**
   —is the preferred method of managing long-term hydrocephalus.
   a. **Ventriculoperitoneal (VP) shunts**
      —are the most commonly used shunts.
   b. **Ventriculoatrial (VA) shunts**
      —with CSF shunted into the right atrium are used when abdominal pathology precludes use of VP shunts.
   c. **Ventriculopleural shunts**
      —are used when other shunts are contraindicated.

C. **Neural tube defects**
   1. The **incidence**
      —is 1/1000 live births, most commonly affecting **white females.**
   2. The **least severe lesion** is **spina bifida occulta,** which is usually asymptomatic and found incidentally on radiograph.
   3. **Myelomeningocele** (MMC)
      a. This is the most common clinically significant lesion.
      b. MMC is a herniation of the spinal cord and nerve roots outside the spinal canal through a defect in the vertebrae.
         —They most commonly occur in the lumbar region.
      c. Presentation ranges from a mild deformity to complete motor and sensory loss.
         —If the hernia sac is ruptured, immediate surgical closure should be performed to prevent infection.

D. **Craniosynostosis**
   —is defined as **premature closure of one or more cranial sutures,** leading to irregular cranial growth.
   1. **Sagittal stenosis**
      —is most common, accounting for 50% of cases.
   2. **Diagnosis**
      —can be made on physical examination, which reveals ridges and decreased mobility along the fused sutures.

3. Surgical repair

—is performed at 3–4 months old, with an operative mortality of less than 1%.

VII. Central Nervous System Infections

A. Spine

1. Epidural abscesses may originate from three potential sources including

—**hematogenous spread** from primary infections at other sites (50% of cases).

—**direct extension** from decubitus ulcers, psoas abscesses, trauma, etc.

—**spinal procedures** such as lumbar puncture, epidural injection, or surgery.

a. Risk factors include

—intravenous (IV) drug use.

—diabetes.

—alcoholism.

—chronic renal failure.

—immunocompromised state.

—epidural anesthesia.

—lumbar puncture.

—surgery.

b. Classic findings include

—back pain.

—fever.

—spinal tenderness.

c. The **most common causative organism** is *Staphylococcus aureus.*

d. Treatment

—involves surgical drainage of the abscess and IV antibiotics.

2. Osteomyelitis

a. This **occurs most commonly** in

—immunocompromised patients.

—the elderly.

—IV drug abusers.

—patients with diabetes or rheumatoid arthritis.

—patients requiring hemodialysis.

b. Patients present with

—fever.

—back pain.

—weight loss.

—neurologic symptoms.

—myelopathy.

c. **Diagnosis** is made by

—clinical examination.

—elevated white blood cell (WBC) count.

—elevated erythrocyte sedimentation rate (ESR).

—characteristic findings on plain films, bone scans, and MRI.

d. The **most common agent** is *S. aureus,* but species can vary based on the source.

e. **Treatment**

—is usually nonoperative with immobilization and IV antibiotics.

3. **Discitis**

a. **Disc space infection**

—can be spontaneous or occur postoperatively.

b. **Patients present**

—primarily with localized pain made worse with movement, often radiating to the hip, lower extremity, groin, abdomen, or perineum.

c. **Examination**

—reveals tenderness to palpation and muscle spasm.

d. **MRI**

—is most useful with involvement in the disc space.

e. Most infections may be **treated** with

—immobilization and IV antibiotics.

—Surgery is indicated for nerve root decompression or abscess drainage.

B. **Cerebral**

1. **Brain abscess**

a. **Risk factors** include

—pulmonary infection.

—bronchiectasis.

—lung abscess/empyema.

—cyanotic heart disease.

—bacterial endocarditis.

—pulmonary AV fistula.

—sinus infections (frontal, middle ear, mastoid).

—immunosuppression.

—penetrating head injury.

—cranial surgery.

b. **Potential sources of infection** include

—hematogenous spread.

—direct extension.

—penetrating head injury.

—cranial procedures.

c. **Streptococcus species are common,** although multiple organisms may frequently be present.

   d. Symptoms
      —are generally related to increased ICP and seizures.
   e. Diagnosis
      (1) Evaluation will show increased WBC, ESR, and C-reactive protein.
      (2) MRI provides better images but CT scans are often diagnostic.
      (3) If possible, a **tissue biopsy** should be obtained to identify the inciting organisms and to rule out potential coexisting lesions (e.g., cystic glioma, metastatic tumor, lymphoma, cysticercosis cyst, infarct, hematoma).
   f. Treatment
      (1) Initial treatment
         —involves administration of broad spectrum antibiotics.
      (2) Antibiotics
         —specific for the organisms should be continued for 6–8 weeks.
      (3) Surgery is indicated for patients with
         —a significant mass effect.
         —lesions near the ventricle.
         —poor neurologic status.
         —abscess progression despite medical therapy.

2. Subdural empyema
   a. This may be secondary to sinusitis, otitis, previous surgery, trauma, or depressed skull fractures.
   b. Treatment
      —involves craniotomy with debridement and IV antibiotics.

VIII. Miscellaneous

A. Epilepsy
   1. The **focus is localized**
      —anatomically by CT and MRI.
      —functionally by electroencephalogram (EEG).
   2. Surgery is indicated for epilepsy
      —that significantly impairs daily function.
      —that is inadequately controlled on medication for at least 1 year.
      —The goal of surgery is to resect the focus of seizure activity.

B. Neurocutaneous disorders (Table 7-7)
   —Hemangioblastomas associated with these disorders may secrete **erythropoietin**.
   —Ten to twenty percent of patients have erythrocytosis.

C. Neurofibromatosis (NFT) type I (von Recklinghausen's disease type I) (see Table 7-7)
   1. The **diagnosis** requires at least 2 of the following:

Table 7-7. Characteristics of Neurocutaneous Disorders

Disorder	Genetics	Clinical Features	Management Considerations
von Hippel-Lindau syndrome	Autosomal dominant, 90% penetrance; involves chromosome 3	Retinal and cerebellar hemangioblastomas; tumors/cysts of kidneys and pancreas; erythrocytosis	Cystic hemangioblastomas may be removed surgically; mural nodules must be removed to prevent recurrence
Neurofibromatosis type I (von Recklinghausen's disease type I)	Autosomal dominant, 100% penetrance; involves chromosome 19	Café-au-lait spots, Lesch nodules, plexiform neurofibromas, axillary freckling, optic gliomas	Focal, symptomatic lesions may be surgically resected; optic gliomas should be followed surgically and resected if symptomatic
Neurofibromatosis type II	Autosomal dominant; involves chromosome 22	Bilateral acoustic neuromas, neurofibromas, optic gliomas, meningiomas, juvenile cataracts	Hearing may be preserved with early removal of acoustic neuromas
Tuberous sclerosis (Bourneville's disease)	Autosomal dominant	Classical presentation is clinical triad of seizures, mental retardation, and adenoma sebaceum. Typical cutaneous lesions: adenoma sebaceum, shagreen patch, ash leaf macules; hamartomas of multiple organ systems	Seizures are treated pharmacologically; resection of the seizure focus may be attempted for intractable disease; paraventricular tumors should be removed if symptomatic

—**café-au-lait spots** (i.e., cutaneous patches of hyperpigmentation)

—**Lesch nodules** (i.e., pigmented hamartomas on the iris).

—**optic gliomas**

—a first-degree relative with the disease

—axillary freckling

—bony defects

2. **Neurofibromas**

—typically present in peripheral nerves.

3. **Plexiform neurofibromas**

—appear as a "bag of worms" in the skin.

D. **Neurofibromatosis type II** (see Table 7-7)

1. The **finding of bilateral vestibular schwannomas** is diagnostic for NFT type II.

2. NFT II can also be **diagnosed** with 2 or more of the following:

—neurofibroma or schwannoma

—meningioma

—glioma

—juvenile cataracts

E. Tuberous sclerosis (Bourneville's disease) (see Table 7-7)

1. The three **typical cutaneous lesions** associated with tuberous sclerosis are

—**adenoma sebaceum** (i.e., angiofibromas that look like facial acne).

—**shagreen patch** (i.e., a hypomelanotic area in the lumbosacral region).

—**ash leaf macules** (i.e., hypopigmented linear macules on the trunk or limbs).

2. **Hamartomas** of the skin, retinae, and other organs are a common finding.

3. **Survival**

—Fifty percent die in childhood.

—Mortality in adulthood is often related to uncontrollable seizures.

Review Test

Directions: Each of the numbered items or incomplete statements in this section is followed by answers or by completions of the statement. Select the ONE lettered answer or completion that is BEST in each case.

1. An elderly man slips in his bathroom and sustains a blow to the head. His wife finds him unconscious and unresponsive. At the hospital, he is diagnosed with an acute subdural hematoma. Which of the following characteristics are most consistent with this diagnosis?

(A) Lucid interval, middle meningeal artery tear, and lenticular shape on computed tomography (CT) scan
(B) "Motor oil" appearance of the hematoma upon removal, low density on CT scan
(C) Hydrocephalus requiring ventriculostomy, blood seen in ventricles on CT scan
(D) Caused by tearing of bridging vessels, crescent shape on CT, intermediate density on CT
(E) Caused by tearing of bridging vessels, lenticular shape on CT, intermediate density on CT

2. A 45-year-old woman presents to your office with complaints of early morning headaches accompanied by vomiting, diplopia, and decreasing visual acuity. Which of the following is the most appropriate next step in the management of this patient?

(A) Prescribe analgesics and antiemetics and tell the patient to come back in 2 weeks
(B) Order an immediate computed tomography (CT) or magnetic resonance imaging (MRI) scan of the patient's head
(C) Refer the patient to a chronic pain management center
(D) Proceed to the operating room for emergent burr hole placement to relieve increased intracranial pressure
(E) Admit the patient to the hospital and follow serial neurologic examinations

3. After a recent office visit for evaluation of headaches accompanied by nausea and vomiting and progressive truncal ataxia, a 4-year-old boy is diagnosed with medulloblastoma. Which of the following statements regarding these tumors is true?

(A) Medulloblastoma is one of the rarer primary brain tumors in children
(B) First line treatment should include surgical debulking with radiation therapy
(C) Chemotherapy with carmustine is effective at inducing remission of medulloblastomas
(D) Most of these tumors arise from the floor of the fourth ventricle
(E) Intracranial spread of these tumors is rare at the time of diagnosis

4. An emaciated, 65-year-old man presents to your office with complaints of progressive motor weakness and recent weight loss. A head computed tomography (CT) scan shows a lesion in the right cerebral hemisphere. Which of the following is the most appropriate next step in this patient's management?

(A) Send him to the operating room for immediate removal of the lesion
(B) Admit him to the hospital for neurologic evaluation and stereotactic biopsy of the lesion
(C) Complete cancer work-up
(D) Admit for CCNU (lomustine) chemotherapy, followed by a course of radiation therapy
(E) Refer him to hospice care

5. A woman brings her 10 year-old son to your office for an annual physical examination. She mentions that her son has von Hippel-Landau disease. Which of the following is characteristic of this disease?

(A) Lesch nodules
(B) Inheritance as an autosomal recessive trait
(C) Bilateral acoustic neuromas
(D) Café-au-lait spots
(E) Cerebellar hemangioblastomas

6. A 46-year-old man presents to the emergency room with the acute onset of severe headache, stiff neck, and photophobia. No neurologic deficits were evident on examination. Head computed tomography (CT) scan obtained in the emergency room shows blood in the basal cisterns. The patient is diagnosed with subarachnoid hemorrhage (SAH). Which of the following statements regarding SAH is true?

(A) Ruptured arteriovenous malformations (AVMs) are the most common cause of nontraumatic SAH in adults

(B) A CT scan is the best radiographic measure for localization of the bleeding lesion

(C) Cerebrospinal fluid xanthochromia is an uncommon finding within 12 hours of SAH

(D) Cerebral aneurysms can be caused by infectious agents

(E) Vasospasm is a greater problem in SAH after a ruptured AVM than after a ruptured cerebral aneurysm

7. A 4-year-old boy is recovering postoperatively from surgical debulking of a medulloblastoma. He begins to experience gradually worsening headaches that are accompanied by nausea and vomiting. Physical examination is notable for papilledema. Which of the following is true about this child's condition?

(A) Computed tomography (CT) scan will most likely show "slit-like" ventricles

(B) This patient probably suffers from communicating hydrocephalus

(C) This condition occurs in about 20% of pediatric patients postoperatively

(D) A ventriculoatrial shunt would be the best choice for treatment of this condition

(E) Dilation of the cerebral aqueduct is one possible cause of this condition

8. A 33-year-old man sustains multiple injuries in a motor vehicle accident. Upon evaluation in the emergency room, the patient is unconscious and is noted to have a blood pressure of 50/30 mm Hg despite administration of 2 L of crystalloid solution. Diagnostic peritoneal lavage is grossly positive. In regards to management of a potential head injury, which of the following strategies would be the most appropriate for this patient?

(A) Emergent laparotomy with immediate postoperative head computed tomography (CT) scan

(B) Immediate head CT scan, followed by emergent laparotomy

(C) Placement of intracranial pressure (ICP) monitor in the emergency room, followed by emergent laparotomy

(D) Placement of ICP monitor after laparotomy if postoperative neurologic examination is abnormal

(E) Placement of ICP monitor intra-operatively during emergent laparotomy

9. A 28-year-old man was severely beaten and thrown to the ground. Upon examination at a local hospital, he was found to have a basilar skull fracture. Which of the following is infrequently associated with basilar skull fractures?

(A) Battle's sign

(B) Periorbital ecchymoses

(C) Cranial nerve (CN) XII injury

(D) Cerebrospinal fluid otorrhea

(E) Hemotympanum

10. A 30-year-old woman has been having trouble getting pregnant and has recently begun to feel as if her vision has worsened. She is also having headaches. A magnetic resonance imaging (MRI) of the head demonstrates an abnormal mass in the sella turcica impinging on the optic chiasm. Which of the following laboratory studies is NOT part of the initial evaluation of this patient?

(A) Thyroid panel [thyroxine (T_4) and thyroid stimulating hormone (TSH)]

(B) Cosyntropin stimulation test

(C) Prolactin level

(D) Estradiol level

(E) Serum ceruloplasmin

Directions: The group of items in this section consists of lettered options followed by a set of numbered items. For each item, select the lettered option(s) that is (are) most closely associated with it. Each lettered option may be selected once, more than once, or not at all.

Questions 11–15

(A) Ependymoma
(B) Oligodendroglioma
(C) Meningioma
(D) Glioblastoma multiforme
(E) Cerebellar astrocytoma
(F) Medulloblastoma
(G) Craniopharyngioma

For each of the following clinical scenarios, select the brain tumor most closely associated.

11. A 5-year-old boy presents with headaches and ataxia, and has a lesion arising from the fourth ventricle on computed tomography (CT) scan. (SELECT 2 TUMORS)

12. A 45-year-old woman with a long history of headaches has a large olfactory groove mass on computed tomography (CT) scan. (SELECT 1 TUMOR)

13. An 8-year-old boy presents with headaches and ataxia, and has a lesion arising from the floor of the fourth ventricle on computed tomography (CT) scan. (SELECT 1 TUMOR)

14. A middle aged man presents with a long history of seizures and a calcified frontal lobe lesion. (SELECT 1 TUMOR)

15. An 8-year-old child presents to the office with visual field deficits, headache, and is found to have an elevated prolactin level upon evaluation. (SELECT 1 TUMOR)

Questions 16–18

(A) von Hippel-Landau disease
(B) Prolactin-secreting adenoma
(C) Neurofibromatosis type II
(D) Growth hormone-secreting adenoma
(E) Cushing's disease
(F) Tuberous sclerosis
(G) Neurofibromatosis type I

For each clinical characteristic listed, select the disorder most closely associated.

16. A 6-year-old boy is found to have pigmented hamartomatous lesions of the iris and an optic glioma upon funduscopic examination. (SELECT 1 CHARACTERISTIC)

17. A 25-year-old woman presents with worsening hearing loss and tinnitus. A computed tomography (CT) scan reveals tumor involvement of cranial nerve VIII bilaterally. (SELECT 1 CHARACTERISTIC)

18. A 25-year-old woman presents with complaints of significant weight gain, amenorrhea, and "purple lines" on her skin. (SELECT 1 CHARACTERISTIC)

Answers and Explanations

1-D. An acute subdural hematoma usually results from tearing of the bridging vessels. The appearance on computed tomography (CT) can be high or intermediate density, and the collection of blood is usually crescent shaped. The symptoms of a lucid interval, lenticular shape on CT, and tearing of the middle meningeal artery is classic for an epidural hematoma. The gross "motor oil" appearance is typical for a chronic subdural hematoma. Hydrocephalus that requires ventriculostomy placement is suggestive of traumatic intraventricular hemorrhage.

2-B. This patient's history is worrisome for an intracranial mass lesion, and she should have a computed tomography (CT) or magnetic resonance imaging (MRI) scan of her head immediately after her history and physical examination. She has symptoms that are suggestive of increased intracranial pressure, which could be due to a mass lesion such as a tumor. Her symptoms could also be caused by hydrocephalus. In either case, imaging will be vital to diagnosis. Ignoring this problem or just treating the symptoms will endanger the patient's life. The patient may need operative intervention, but surgery should wait until the entity causing her symptoms is better characterized.

3-B. The treatment of choice for medulloblastomas is surgical debulking and radiation therapy, which results in a 5-year survival of 56%. Chemotherapy with carmustine is sometimes used in relapse, but is ineffective as an initial treatment modality. Medulloblastomas are the most common brain tumors in children. They are associated with the roof of the fourth ventricle, not the floor. Subarachnoid spread is seen in 35% of cases at the time of diagnosis.

4-C. While it is possible that this patient has a primary brain tumor, his old age and significant weight loss should raise the possibility of metastatic disease. Before any treatment modality is selected, a complete metastatic work-up should be performed. The work-up should include a thorough history and physical examination (rectal examination is important here); complete blood count; serum chemistries; liver function tests; carcinoembryonic antigen (CEA); cancer antigen 125 test (CA-125); chest radiograph; computed tomography (CT) scan of chest, abdomen, and pelvis; and mammogram to identify the potential primary tumor.

5-E. Associated with retinal and cerebellar hemangioblastomas, von Hippel-Landau disease is inherited as an autosomal dominant trait. This disease may also be associated with elevated erythropoietin production, leading to erythrocytosis. Lesch nodules, pigmented hamartomas on the iris, are characteristic of neurofibromatosis. Café-au-lait spots and bilateral acoustic neuromas are associated with neurofibromatosis type I and II, respectively.

6-D. About 80% of nontraumatic subarachnoid hemorrhage (SAH) in adults is caused by ruptured cerebral aneurysms. Cerebral angiography is generally considered the best radiographic technique for localizing the bleeding lesion. In addition to blood on a computed tomography (CT) scan, cerebrospinal fluid xanthochromia is also diagnostic for SAH and is a common finding within 12 hours of rupture from an SAH. Aneurysms can be caused by infectious agents as well. When this is the case, they are referred to as mycotic aneurysms. Postbleed vasospasm is a much greater problem in ruptured aneurysms than in ruptured arteriovenous malformations (AVMs). In fact, vasospasm is rare in ruptured AVMs.

7-C. Hydrocephalus is an abnormal excess of cerebrospinal fluid (CSF) associated with dilation of the ventricular system. If CSF excess is caused by a blockage in the intracranial CSF pathways, it is referred to as noncommunicating hydrocephalus. Postoperatively, 20% of pediatric patients may develop noncommunicating hydrocephalus. This can be from stenosis of the cerebral aqueduct. The treatment of choice is a ventriculoperitoneal shunt. Ventriculoatrial shunts are used if ventriculoperitoneal shunts are not feasible.

8-E. This is a common dilemma in patients sustaining multiple injuries including a presumed head injury after a motor vehicle accident. In a severely hypotensive patient not responding to initial resuscitative measures with a grossly positive peritoneal lavage, the primary goal of therapy should be rapid identification and control of sources of life-threatening hemorrhage. Thus emergent laparotomy is essential in this patient. When unable to adequately evaluate the patient for a suspected head injury either by performing a neurologic examination in the emergency room or performing a head computed tomography (CT) scan, an intracranial pressure (ICP) monitor should be placed immediately without delaying other treatment measures (i.e., laparotomy). Thus, placement of the ICP monitor intraoperatively simultaneously with performance of the laparotomy would be most appropriate in this patient.

9-C. Cranial nerve (CN) XII is not damaged in basilar skull fractures. The nerves most often damaged in this sort of injury are CN I, VII, and VIII. The other signs of basilar skull fractures include hemotympanum, cerebrospinal fluid otorrhea or rhinorrhea, Battle's sign (postauricular ecchymoses), and periorbital ecchymoses (raccoon eyes). Many basilar skull fractures do not require treatment.

10-E. This woman's history is suggestive of a pituitary adenoma. After a thorough history and physical examination, laboratory studies to assess her neuroendocrine function are essential. Visual field testing should also be performed. The most common visual field deficit seen in patients with pituitary adenomas is bitemporal hemianopsia. The physician should also take a good family history to search for evidence of multiple endocrine neoplasia (MEN) I. Ceruloplasmin levels are not directly affected by lesions in the pituitary and are of no use in the work-up of these patients.

11-F or A. The boy in the question has a classic presentation of a mass located in the fourth ventricle. However, both medulloblastoma and ependymoma are possibilities. A definitive answer can only be made based on the histology of the resected tumor.

12-C. Meningiomas are slow growing tumors that often present with complaints of chronic headache. The olfactory groove is a common location for meningiomas.

13-A. This child also has a classic presentation of a fourth ventricle mass. However, because this mass is seen to be arising from the floor of the ventricle, ependymoma is most likely. Medulloblastomas more commonly arise from the roof of the ventricle. Histology will still make the final diagnosis.

14-B. Patients with oligodendrogliomas classically present with a long history of seizures. These tumors are often calcified on computed tomography (CT) scan and most commonly occur in the frontal lobe.

15-G. Craniopharyngiomas are most common in children and present with symptoms of headache, visual field deficits, and endocrine abnormalities. This is because of their location in the suprasellar region in close proximity to the pituitary and optic chiasm.

16-G. Lesch nodules (pigmented hamartomas of the iris) and optic gliomas are two of the criteria that can be used to diagnose neurofibromatosis type I. Other characteristics include plexiform neurofibromas and autosomal dominant inheritance.

17-C. The finding of bilateral vestibular schwannomas involving cranial nerve VIII is considered diagnostic for neurofibromatosis type II.

18-E. These findings are suggestive of hypercortisolism. This may be secondary to a number of sources including adrenal tumors, exogenous steroid use, pituitary tumors, and malignancies at other sites (e.g., small cell carcinoma of the lung). Among the choices, Cushing's disease defined as hypercortisolism secondary to an adrenocorticotropic hormone (ACTH)-producing pituitary adenoma, is the most likely diagnosis.

8

Ophthalmology

Ken A. Barba

I. Functional Anatomy (Figures 8.1 and 8.2)

A. Anterior structures that can be viewed grossly or with a slit lamp include the

—lids.

—cornea.

—conjunctiva.

—sclera.

—iris.

—pupil.

—anterior chamber.

—lens.

B. Posterior structures that are seen by direct ophthalmoscopy are the

—vitreous humor.

—retina.

—optic nerve.

C. Cranial nerve (CN) III (i.e., oculomotor) innervates

—the **superior, medial,** and **inferior recti.**

—the **inferior oblique and levator palpebral** (i.e., upper eyelid) muscles.

D. CN IV (i.e., trochlear) innervates

—the **superior oblique.**

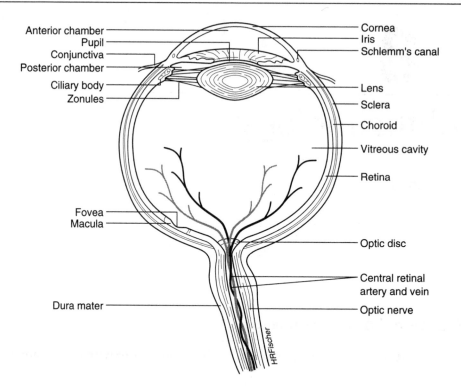

Figure 8.1. Anatomy of the eye. (Adapted with permission from Berson FG: *Basic Ophthalmology for Medical Students and Primary Care Residents,* 6th ed. San Francisco, American Academy of Ophthalmology, 1993, p 4.)

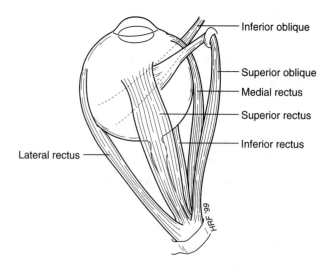

Figure 8.2. Extraocular muscles. (Adapted with permission from Berson FG: *Basic Ophthalmology for Medical Students and Primary Care Residents,* 6th ed. San Francisco, American Academy of Ophthalmology, 1993, p 5.)

E. CN VI (i.e., abducens) innervates

—the **lateral rectus.**

II. Infectious and Inflammatory Disorders (Tables 8-1 and 8-2)

A. Conjunctivitis

   1. **Viruses** are by far the **most common cause.**

      a. **Signs and symptoms** include

         —**watery discharge.**

         —redness.

         —normal or mildly decreased vision.

         —mild irritation.

      b. The **course** is generally benign and no specific treatment is required.

         —Conjunctivitis, however, is **very contagious.**

   2. **Bacterial infection** is marked by **purulent discharge,** redness, normal or mildly decreased vision, and mild to moderate discomfort.

      a. **Treatment** is with topical antibiotics.

      b. A **Gram stain** will help rule out **gonococcal** infection with identification of **gram-negative diplococci** within white blood cells.

         —Gonococcal infection requires **systemic and topical treatment** with close ophthalmologic follow-up.

   3. The hallmark of **allergic conjunctivitis** is **itching** with a mucinous and stringy discharge.

   4. **Neonatal conjunctivitis** can be caused by either

      —*Chlamydia* species (5–14 days after birth).

      —**gonococci** (1–3 days after birth).

   5. A **pterygium** is a benign, fleshy, wedge-shaped conjunctival overgrowth.

      —It should not be confused with infectious or inflammatory conjunctivitis.

B. Keratitis (i.e., inflamed cornea)

   1. **Herpes simplex**

      —causes a dendritic corneal epithelial defect.

      a. It is seen best with fluorescein dye and blue light.

      b. Topical steroids are contraindicated.

   2. **Herpes zoster ophthalmicus** (i.e., shingles)

      —occurs along the ophthalmic division of the trigeminal nerve (CN V).

      a. Fifty percent of patients with shingles develop ocular involvement.

      b. Those with lesions on the tip of the nose (i.e., **Hutchinson sign**) are at greater risk of developing ocular complications.

C. Hordeolum (i.e., stye)

   —is an acute, tender, erythematous infection of an eyelash follicle usually caused by *Staphylococcus* species.

Table 8-1. Signs of Red Eye

Sign	Referral Advisable if Present	Acute Glaucoma	Acute Iridocyclitis	Keratitis	Conjunctivitis		
					Bacterial	Viral	Allergic
Ciliary flush	Yes	1	2	3	0	0	0
Conjunctival hyperemia	No	2	2	2	3	2	1
Corneal opacification	Yes	3	0	1 to 3	0	0 or 1	0
Corneal epithelial disruption	Yes	0	0	1 to 3	0	0 or 1	0
Pupillary abnormalities	Yes	Mid-dilated, nonreactive	Small, may be irregular	Normal or small	0	0	0
Shallow anterior chamber depth	Yes	3	0	0	0	0	0
Elevated intraocular pressure	Yes	3	-2 to $+1$	0	0	0	0
Proptosis	Yes	0	0	0	0	0	0
Discharge	No	0	0	Sometimes	2 or 3	2	1
Preauricular lymph-node enlargement	No	0	0	0	0	1	0

Note: The range of severity of the sign is indicated by -2 (subnormal) to 0 (absent) to 3 (severe). (Reprinted with permission from Berson FG: *Basic Ophthalmology for Medical Students and Primary Care Residents*, 6th ed. San Francisco, American Academy of Ophthalmology, 1993, p 64.)

Table 8-2. Symptoms of Red Eye

Symptom	Referral Advisable if Present	Acute Glaucoma	Acute Iridocyclitis	Keratitis	Conjunctivitis		
					Bacterial	Viral	Allergic
Blurred vision	Yes	3	1 to 2	3	0	0	0
Pain	Yes	2 to 3	2	2	0	0	0
Photophobia	Yes	1	3	3	0	0	0
Colored halos	Yes	2	0	0	0	0	0
Exudation	No	0	0	0 to 3	3	2	1
Itching	No	0	0	0	0	0	2 to 3

Note: The range of severity of the sign is indicated by 0 (absent) to 3 (severe).
(Reprinted with permission from Berson FG: *Basic Ophthalmology for Medical Students and Primary Care Residents*, 6th ed. San Francisco, American Academy of Ophthalmology, 1993, p 65.)

—is effectively treated with hot packs.

D. Chalazion

—is a chronic, nontender, round firm granuloma.

—is generally treated with hot packs and, occasionally, incision and drainage.

E. Preseptal cellulitis

—is an infection of the eyelids or skin around the eyes.

—is characterized by periocular redness, swelling, warmth, or tenderness.

F. Orbital cellulitis

—is infection in the orbit or eye socket.

1. Signs and symptoms may include

—**restricted and painful eye movements.**

—decreased vision.

—**proptosis** (bulging eye).

—a **relative afferent pupillary defect,** or Marcus Gunn pupil (seen with the swinging flashlight test).

2. Complications may include

—meningitis.

—brain abscess.

—cavernous sinus thrombosis.

—subperiosteal abscess.

G. Episcleritis

—is a benign, self-limited, unilateral, sectoral redness of the eye that needs no specific treatment.

H. Scleritis

—is a **diffuse inflammation** of the scleral tissue.

1. Signs and symptoms include

—**pain.**

—**tenderness.**

—redness.

—normal vision.

2. An ophthalmologic evaluation is indicated because of the potential for associated systemic disease (e.g., rheumatoid arthritis, systemic lupus erythematosus).

I. Uveitis

—is inflammation of any pigmented structure of the eye, including iris (i.e., **iritis**), ciliary body (i.e., **cyclitis**), and choroid (i.e., **choroiditis**).

1. Iritis or iridocyclitis is

—usually unilateral.

—associated with mild to moderate **pain, photophobia,** mild decrease in vision, and redness.

2. This **inflammation may be** secondary to trauma, infection, or an associated systemic disease, or it may be idiopathic.

3. **Management should include**

—a referral for an ophthalmologic evaluation and treatment.

J. Cytomegalovirus (CMV) retinitis

—is associated with immunocompromised states such as acquired immunodeficiency syndrome (AIDS).

1. The infected retina reveals a zone of white and fluffy necrosis with hemorrhages and a distinct border of normal retina.

2. CMV generally occurs with CD4 counts less than 50.

III. Neuro-ophthalmology

A. Visual field defects (Figure 8.3)

1. **Lesions from the retina** to the optic chiasm will produce defects only in one eye.

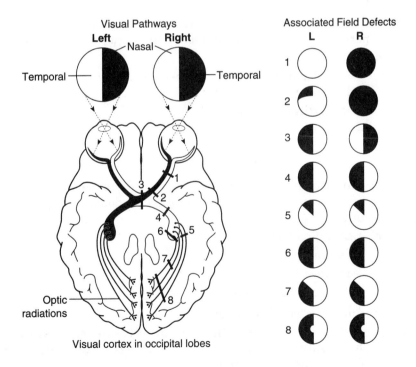

Figure 8.3. Visual field defects by lesion location. (Adapted with permission from Berson FG: *Basic Ophthalmology for Medical Students and Primary Care Residents,* 6th ed. San Francisco, American Academy of Ophthalmology, 1993, p 116.)

2. **Lesions from the optic chiasm** to the occipital cortex result in bilateral defects.

3. **Bitemporal hemianopia**
    a. **This condition is characterized by both**
        —loss of the **right half** of vision in the **right eye.**
        —loss of the **left half** of vision in the **left eye.**
    b. Bitemporal hemianopia is **caused by lesions of the optic chiasm,** such as
        —pituitary tumors.
        —meningiomas.
        —gliomas.
        —craniopharyngiomas.

4. **Homonymous hemianopias**
    —(i.e., loss of right half of vision for the right and left eyes) result from lesions posterior to the chiasm, most commonly **strokes.**

5. **Confrontational visual field testing**
    —may detect these defects.

B. **Cranial nerve palsies**

1. **Oculomotor nerve (CN III) paresis** results in
    —ipsilateral **ptosis** (i.e., droopy lid) from loss of levator palpebral function.
    —**diplopia** with the eye in a **"down and out"** position from loss of superior, inferior, and medial recti, and inferior oblique muscle function.
    a. **With normal pupils**
        —consider microvascular disease secondary to hypertension or diabetes as potential causes.
    b. **With a dilated pupil**
        —consider aneurysm or extradural hematoma with temporal lobe herniation.

2. **Trochlear nerve (CN IV) paresis**
    a. Trochlear nerve paresis **causes** a loss of superior oblique function, which results in **vertical diplopia** (i.e., double images on top of each other).
    b. **Etiologies** include
        —trauma.
        —microvascular disease.
        —congenital anomalies.

3. **Abducens (CN VI) paresis**
    a. Abducens paresis **inhibits** lateral rectus function, which results in **horizontal diplopia** (i.e., double images side by side). The affected eye is turned in (esotropic).
    b. **Etiologies** include
        —microvascular disease.
        —**acoustic neuromas.**

—increased intracranial pressure.

—basilar skull fractures.

—nasopharyngeal tumors.

—aneurysms (rare).

4. **Examine extraocular muscles** with an "H" pattern to isolate each muscle.

C. **Giant cell arteritis** (i.e., temporal arteritis)

—may cause **vision loss** due to arteritic ischemic optic neuropathy.

1. **Other symptoms** may include

—headache.

—weight loss.

—night sweats, fever, chills.

—jaw claudication.

—myalgias.

—arthralgias.

2. **This disease** generally occurs in the elderly and is uncommon in African Americans.

3. **Elevations in erythrocyte sedimentation rate** and C reactive protein may be suggestive.

—Definitive diagnosis requires **temporal artery biopsy.**

D. **Horner syndrome**

—is the triad of **ptosis** (i.e., droopy lid), **miosis** (i.e., small pupil), and **anhydrosis** (i.e., decreased sweat production).

1. **Signs occur** ipsilateral to the lesions, causing injury to sympathetic nerve fibers.

2. **Etiologies** include

—Pancoast's tumor at the apex of the lung.

—carotid aneurysms.

—neck lesions.

—a history of neck trauma or surgery.

E. **Optic neuritis** (i.e., papillitis)

1. **Symptoms** include

—**unilateral** decrease in vision.

—pain with eye movement.

2. **There may be** a **relative afferent pupillary defect** and optic nerve head swelling.

3. A **magnetic resonance imaging (MRI) scan**

—of the brain may be indicated to rule out **multiple sclerosis.**

4. **Internuclear ophthalmoplegia**

—may also be seen with multiple sclerosis.

  a. This is secondary to lesions in the medial longitudinal fasciculus.

  b. Signs include defective a*d*duction of the ipsilaterally affected eye with normal a*b*duction and normal convergence.

F. Nystagmus

  1. The **pendular type**

   —reveals the same speed in both directions, as seen with congenitally poor vision.

  2. Jerk nystagmus

   —has a slow and fast phase.

   a. This may be benign, as seen with **end-gaze and with some drugs** (e.g., phenytoin, barbiturates).

   b. This may also indicate a **vestibular disorder** (e.g., tumors, multiple sclerosis).

  3. Downbeat nystagmus

   —is suggestive of Arnold-Chiari malformation.

  4. Upbeat nystagmus

   —suggests posterior fossa lesions or certain drugs (e.g., phenytoin).

G. Papilledema

  —is **bilateral** optic nerve swelling from **increased intracranial pressure.**

  1. Vision is usually normal or mildly decreased.

  2. On examination, the optic disc has blurred margins, hemorrhages, and engorged veins.

  3. It is **initially important** to rule out malignant hypertension as a potential cause.

  4. Subsequent evaluation

   —for a space-occupying lesion of the brain should be performed [e.g., computed tomography (CT) or MRI].

  5. The **diagnosis of pseudotumor cerebri** (benign intracranial hypertension)

   —should be considered with normal blood pressure and CT or MRI.

IV. Trauma

A. Corneal abrasion

  —is **best seen with fluorescein dye** and a cobalt blue light (e.g., **Wood's lamp** or slit lamp).

  1. Symptoms include

   —sensation of a foreign body.

   —redness.

   —mild or moderate pain.

      —mild or moderate decrease in vision.

      —photophobia.

   2. Treatment includes antibiotic as either

      —frequent topical drops.

      —ointment with a patch and daily follow-up until healing is complete.

B. Foreign bodies

   1. Most foreign bodies within the eye are metallic in origin.

   2. They can generally be removed under a slit lamp, frequently with a tuberculin syringe.

      —An eye patch is placed after the object is removed.

C. Orbital wall fracture

   1. Medial wall fracture

      —may result in periocular subcutaneous emphysema.

   2. Orbital floor fractures

      —may cause restricted upgaze from inferior rectus and orbital contents herniating into the maxillary sinus, causing **diplopia.**

D. Chemical injury

      —requires **irrigating** the eye with normal saline until an ophthalmologic evaluation can be performed.

E. Hyphema

      —is layered blood in the anterior chamber, which may result from blunt trauma.

      —requires ophthalmologic evaluation because re-bleeding and glaucoma may occur.

F. Ruptured eyeball or open globe injury

   1. This disorder is **characterized by**

      —poor vision.

      —extensive subconjunctival hemorrhage.

      —hyphema.

      —obvious penetrating injury.

   2. Treatment

      —Place a protective metal shield, cup, or anything sturdy over the eye and obtain immediate ophthalmologic consultation.

V. Retinal Lesions

A. Age-related macular degeneration

      —causes a **central scotoma (i.e., blind spot).**

      —is the leading cause of blindness in people over 60 years old.

B. **Central retinal artery occlusion**

1. This **occlusion causes** sudden, painless, monocular loss of vision.

2. It **may be caused by** an embolic event from carotid artery or heart valve disease.

3. **Examination may reveal**

—poor vision.

—relative afferent pupillary defect.

—a pale retina with a **cherry red spot at the fovea.**

C. **Central retinal vein occlusion**

1. This **type of occlusion** also causes sudden, painless, monocular loss of vision.

2. It may be **associated** with **hypertension.**

3. **Examination may reveal**

—poor vision.

—relative afferent pupillary defect.

—dramatic appearance to the retina with many **retinal hemorrhages,** cotton wool spots, and engorged vessels.

D. **Retinal detachment**

1. **Symptoms** may include

—sensations of flashers, floaters, and cobwebs.

—a shade or curtain seemingly coming down over a field of vision.

2. **Emergent surgical intervention is indicated.**

E. **Diabetes**

1. **Background diabetic retinopathy** includes

—microaneurysms.

—dot, blot, or flame hemorrhages.

—hard exudates.

—cotton wool spots.

2. **Proliferative diabetic retinopathy** may include

—any or all of the background characteristics.

—neovascularization of the optic disc, retina, or iris.

a. This type of diabetic retinopathy can result in vitreous hemorrhage.

b. This process can be effectively treated with laser surgery.

F. **Hypertensive retinopathy**

1. This **condition is marked by**

—thin retinal vessels.

—arteriovenous nicking.

—copper wiring.

—hard exudates.

—flame hemorrhages.

2. Malignant hypertension

—includes all of these findings, in addition to papilledema.

G. Retinopathy of prematurity may affect

—newborns born under 36 weeks gestation or who weigh less than 1500 g and require supplemental oxygen support.

VI. Miscellaneous

A. Cataract

1. Symptomatic cataracts

—are an **opacity of the lens** that result in impaired vision.

—**Cataract extraction** with artificial intraocular lens implantation may be indicated.

2. Congenital cataract

—should be immediately evaluated for possible extraction, because it may result in lack of visual development in children.

B. Arcus senilis

—is a peripheral corneal whitening, which is usually age-related but may rarely be associated with dyslipoproteinemia.

C. Kayser-Fleischer ring

—is a brown deposition of copper in the peripheral cornea associated with Wilson's disease (i.e., hepatolenticular degeneration).

D. Glaucoma

1. Progressive optic nerve atrophy

—is associated with key risk factors.

  a. **Increased intraocular pressure** (normal 10–21 mm Hg) may be identified with a tonometer.

  b. An **increased cup to disc ratio** (normal is less than 40% cup) may be seen on direct ophthalmoscopic examination.

  c. **Characteristic visual field defects** may be seen on automated visual field tests.

  d. A **family history** of glaucoma may also be present.

2. Open angle glaucoma

  a. **This type of glaucoma** is by far the most common type. It is **painless,** usually bilateral, occurs most often in adults, and is usually insidious in nature.

  b. Except for **optic nerve atrophy,** the eyes look healthy, with good central vision.

  c. **Advanced disease results** in loss of peripheral vision, or "**tunnel vision.**"

  d. **Treatment may include**

—topical medications.

—laser procedures.

—surgery.

3. **Angle closure glaucoma**

—is rare but may be dramatic and devastating.

a. **This type of glaucoma is marked by**

—acute onset of **pain.**

—**decreased vision** with "halos."

—nausea and vomiting.

—redness.

—corneal edema that causes an irregular light reflex.

—a fixed nonreactive pupil in a mid-dilated position.

b. This is usually a **unilateral** process.

c. **Intraocular pressure** may be 50 mm Hg or greater.

d. **Treatment**

(1) Try to **lower the eye pressure** with topical glaucoma drops (e.g., timolol, dorzolamide, apraclonidine, pilocarpine).

(2) Consider **systemic agents** (e.g., acetazolamide, mannitol) to help lower pressure and analgesics for **pain.**

(3) Perform a **laser procedure or surgery** to place a hole in the iris to allow the built up aqueous fluid to gain access to the trabecular meshwork.

E. **Refractive error**

—is the most common cause of correctable decrease in vision.

1. **"Sightedness"**

a. **Myopia** is "near-sightedness."

b. **Hyperopia** is "far-sightedness."

c. People in either group may need glasses for both near and distance vision.

2. **Presbyopia**

—is the age-related loss of the ability to accommodate, causing an inability to see near objects with distance corrective lenses.

—Bifocals are often required in this situation.

3. **Astigmatism**

—describes a nonuniform shape to the cornea (i.e., like the surface of a football instead of the surface of a basketball).

F. **Strabismus**

—is a misalignment of the eyes.

1. The **eyes may be turned**

—in (i.e., esotropia).

—out (i.e., exotropia).

—up (i.e., hypertropia).

—down (i.e., hypotropia).

   a. In children, one must be concerned with the possibility of **amblyopia** (i.e., potentially **permanent visual loss** as a result of suppressing the turned-in eye).

   b. Children may require

      —glasses.

      —patching therapy.

      —surgery.

      —any combination thereof.

   c. As an acquired condition in adults the main complaint may be **diplopia,** although cranial nerve palsies (CN III, IV, or VI) may be present.

G. Tumors

1. Melanoma

—is the most common primary intraocular tumor in adults.

2. Metastatic lesions

—are the most common malignant tumor in eyes of adults.

   a. Metastatic lung carcinomas are the most common lesions in men.

   b. Metastatic breast carcinomas are the most common lesions in women.

3. Retinoblastoma

—is the most common intraocular malignancy in **children.**

   a. Leukocoria (white pupil/no red reflex) is frequently present.

   b. This requires immediate ophthalmologic consultation for evaluation and treatment.

Review Test

Directions: Each of the numbered items or incomplete statements in this section is followed by answers or by completions of the statement. Select the ONE lettered answer or completion that is BEST in each case.

1. A 24-year-old man presents with a 1–2 day history of right eye redness, purulent discharge, mild blurring of vision, and mild pain. Examination reveals acuity of 20/25 right and 20/20 left, right conjunctival edema, injection, a clear cornea, and copious creamy purulent discharge. Which of the following would be inappropriate in the management of this patient?

(A) Obtain ophthalmology consultation
(B) Give topical antibiotics with outpatient follow-up
(C) Perform a Gram stain on the discharge
(D) Obtain a thorough sexual history
(E) Initiate appropriate systemic therapy

2. The parents of a 2-year-old child are concerned about the appearance of the child's eye turning inward. The child is otherwise healthy and without symptoms. Which of the following is an inappropriate statement regarding the management of this patient?

(A) If untreated, there is a possibility the vision could be permanently affected
(B) The child may simply need glasses to correct this defect
(C) The child should probably see an ophthalmologist for evaluation
(D) It may be normal at this age, because the visual system is not completely developed
(E) The child may some day require surgery for this problem

3. A 67-year-old woman gives a history of waking with a red eye. She reports a history of taking drops for glaucoma. There is some associated tearing. Examination reveals acuity of 20/25 in both eyes. Which of the following is the most likely diagnosis?

(A) Bacterial conjunctivitis
(B) Pterygium
(C) Viral conjunctivitis
(D) Acute angle closure glaucoma
(E) Corneal abrasion

4. A 61-year-old man presents with a recent history of headaches. Examination reveals papilledema. Which of the following is the next most appropriate step?

(A) Computed tomography (CT) scan of the head
(B) Check blood pressure
(C) Lumbar puncture
(D) Neurosurgical consult
(E) Cerebral angiogram

5. A 68-year-old man presents to the Veterans Administration (VA) general medicine clinic with a 1-day history of significant loss of vision of his right eye. He denies any pain. He has a history of hypertension, insulin-requiring diabetes, and coronary artery disease. Your examination reveals visual acuity of 20/400 right and 20/25 left and a relative afferent pupillary defect of the right eye. The rest of anterior portion of the eye appears to be unremarkable. A dilated fundoscopic examination shows multiple hemorrhages in every retinal quadrant, cotton wool spots, and fat tortuous blood vessels in the right eye. The left eye demonstrated a few microaneurysms and a couple of dot and blot hemorrhages. Which of the following is the most likely diagnosis?

(A) Central retinal vein occlusion
(B) Central retinal artery occlusion
(C) Advanced diabetic retinopathy
(D) Hypertensive retinopathy
(E) Retinal detachment

6. A 22-year-old man is a victim of an alleged assault and is examined in the emergency department. He has multiple contusions and abrasions on the head. He denies any significant change in his visual acuity, but says he sees two of everything, one on top of the other, especially when he tries to look up. Which of the following is most likely to be revealed on radiologic imaging?

(A) Extradural hematoma
(B) Subarachnoid hemorrhage
(C) Brainstem hemorrhage
(D) Open globe injury
(E) Orbital floor fracture

Answers and Explanations

1-B. Gonococcal conjunctivitis may have a hyperacute onset and cause excessive purulent discharge. This requires both topical and systemic treatment, with close ophthalmologic evaluation as an **inpatient.** Outpatient management would be inappropriate in this setting. A thorough history regarding the patient's sexual partners should be obtained in this setting. Notification of the local health department regarding potential contacts is required to allow for appropriate treatment of infected individuals and for prevention of further spread. In the setting of gonococcal conjunctivitis, patients should also be treated for potential *Chlamydia* infection as well. A Gram stain is frequently useful for identification of the causative organism.

2-D. Beyond 2–4 months of age, children should maintain the alignment of their eyes. A 2-year-old needs to be evaluated for strabismus and amblyopia (i.e., decreased vision due to suppression of a healthy eye). Evaluation by an ophthalmologist is essential because of the potential risk of permanent visual changes. Treatment options include glasses, patching, and surgery.

3-C. The signs and symptoms described fit most with viral conjunctivitis, or "pink eye." Bacterial infection usually causes purulence. Pterygium is a benign, chronic, conjunctival overgrowth onto the cornea that is not associated with such symptoms. Angle closure glaucoma results in pain and decreased vision. Abrasions generally cause pain and a sensation of a foreign body.

4-B. The most appropriate initial step in the evaluation would be to check the patient's blood pressure to rule out malignant hypertension as a potential cause of these signs and symptoms. If the blood pressure is normal, evaluation for a space-occupying lesion of the brain should be performed. Such lesions can be identified on head computed tomography (CT) scan. Until a definitive diagnosis is made with imaging studies [e.g., CT or magnetic resonance imaging (MRI)], lumbar puncture, neurosurgical consultation, or cerebral angiography are not necessary at this point.

5-A. Central retinal vein occlusion causes dramatic retinal findings such as multiple retinal hemorrhages, cotton wool spots, and dilated tortuous blood vessels, in contrast to more subtle retinal changes associated with central retinal artery occlusion. It would be very unusual to have such asymmetric distribution with alterations in only one eye with diabetic or hypertensive retinopathy. Retinal detachment is often unilateral but is not characterized by the findings described.

6-E. Temporal lobe herniation would be more likely to result in oculomotor (CN III) palsy, causing ptosis, lack of movement medially as well as upward, and possible pupillary involvement. Subarachnoid and brainstem hemorrhages are unlikely to cause these findings. A ruptured eyeball usually involves decreased vision, pupil abnormalities, subconjunctival hemorrhage, and hyphema (i.e., layered blood in anterior chamber). The signs and symptoms described are characteristic for an orbital floor fracture with restriction in upgaze caused by entrapment of inferior orbital contents (including the inferior rectus muscle) in the maxillary sinus.

Comprehensive Examination

Directions: Each of the numbered items or incomplete statements in this section is followed by answers or by completions of the statement. Select the ONE lettered answer or completion that is BEST in each case.

1. A 55-year-old, male smoker with a history of hypertension presents to the emergency room with acute onset chest pain over the left sternal border. Electrocardiogram (ECG) reveals ST segment elevation in leads V_1–V_4. The patient experiences minimal relief of his chest pain despite administration of nitrates, morphine sulfate, oxygen, and aspirin. While in the emergency room, the patient acutely develops severe shortness of breath and on physical examination he is noted to have a diastolic murmur at the left midclavicular line in the fifth intercostal space. Immediate cardiac catheterization reveals occlusion of the left anterior descending artery (LAD) and severe mitral regurgitation. Which of the following is the most appropriate management strategy in this patient?

(A) Angioplasty of the LAD followed by mitral valve replacement
(B) Immediate surgical bypass of the LAD with papillary muscle repair
(C) Administration of tissue plasminogen activator and coronary artery bypass grafting if the patient does not improve
(D) Angioplasty of the LAD and repeat catheterization if mitral regurgitation does not improve
(E) Immediate surgical bypass of the LAD and mitral valve replacement

2. A 3-year-old child presents with fatigue and anemia. The child's mother reports dark stools and that the child is otherwise healthy. Physical examination is significant only for guaiac-positive stool. Hematocrit is 28%. A colonoscopy is performed and reveals normal colonic mucosa to the level of the cecum. Which of the following is the most likely diagnosis?

(A) Intussusception
(B) Appendicitis
(C) Meconium ileus
(D) Meckel diverticulum
(E) Anal fissure

3. A 52-year-old woman presents with a 24-hour complaint of drooling on herself from the left side of her mouth, a crooked smile, and a sensation of a film over her left eye. She has a past medical history of hypertension and is on a β blocker. She has never had these symptoms before. On physical examination she is noted to have a left facial nerve weakness in all branches. Which of the following would be most appropriate in the initial diagnosis and management of this patient?

(A) Electroneurography of the facial nerve
(B) Head and neck computed tomography (CT) scan
(C) Oral steroid administration
(D) Antibacterial agent administration
(E) Administration of heparin

4. A 6-year-old girl presents to the emergency room after having fallen off her bicycle. She is stable but her right arm hurts her. She has no other injuries. Anterior-posterior and lateral films reveal a supracondylar humerus fracture. Which of the following is a common complication that may develop in this patient?

(A) Acute respiratory distress syndrome (ARDS)
(B) Volkmann's contracture
(C) Skin breakdown
(D) Avascular necrosis of the olecranon
(E) Growth arrest

5. A 55-year-old man with a 3-month history of atrial fibrillation presents with a cold, pulseless right lower extremity. He complains of right leg paresthesia and he is unable to dorsiflex his toes. He undergoes successful popliteal embolectomy with return of pedal pulses, but postoperatively he is still unable to dorsiflex his toes. Which of the following is the next step in the management of this patient?

(A) Elevation of right leg
(B) Repeat embolectomy
(C) Immediate fasciotomy
(D) Application of a posterior splint
(E) Electromyography

6. An active, otherwise healthy, 75-year-old woman was sent to her orthopedist with complaints of intermittent right hip pain over the last 2–3 years. She has no other joint complaints and no constitutional symptoms. She walks 2–3 miles a day and does not require an assist device for ambulating. Pain increases with activity. Work-up includes normal lab results. Radiographs show joint space narrowing with some osteophyte formation on the superior edge of the acetabulum of the right hip. Which of the following is the most appropriate next step in the management of this patient?

(A) Elective total hip replacement
(B) Nonsteroidal anti-inflammatory drugs (NSAIDs), physical therapy, and a cane
(C) Steroid injections into the hip to reduce pain and inflammation
(D) Proximal femoral osteotomy to improve weight bearing
(E) Magnetic resonance imaging (MRI) to rule out malignancy

7. You are called to the pediatric intensive care unit to evaluate a 2-month-old child with intermittent stridor and respiratory distress. The infant's stridor is worse in the supine position. The infant is not cyanotic and has experienced no apneic episodes, and oxygen saturations have always remained greater than 98% on room air. The child has no other congenital problems and is otherwise healthy. The infant has not required intubation. Which of the following would be the most appropriate advice for the parents of this child?

(A) Child may be discharged home and will improve
(B) Child will require long-term hospitalization
(C) Child will require a tracheostomy for airway protection
(D) Child will need to be treated for an infection
(E) Child will require an upper gastrointestinal series to rule out tracheoesophageal fistula

8. A 37-year-old woman presents to the office with complaints of intermittent palpitations and mild dyspnea on exertion. Chest radiograph reveals an enlarged cardiac shadow. Chest computed tomography (CT) scan reveals a 7-cm cystic mass adjacent to the heart at the cardiophrenic angle on the right. Which of the following is the most likely diagnosis in this patient?

(A) Bronchogenic cyst
(B) Esophageal duplication cyst
(C) Pericardial cyst
(D) Pulmonary sequestration
(E) Cystic bronchogenic carcinoma

9. A 1-year-old boy presents to the clinic with a small erythematous lesion on his neck just anterior to the right sternocleidomastoid muscle. The lesion is noted to be draining purulent material from a small central sinus. The mother states that this is the third time that this has occurred despite antibiotic treatment with each episode. Each time the infection has occurred in the same location. Which of the following is an appropriate statement regarding the most likely etiology of this lesion?

(A) The sinus may communicate with the external auditory meatus
(B) The sinus may communicate with the tonsillar fossa
(C) The sinus likely contains thyroid tissue
(D) The lesion is likely associated with an underlying malignancy
(E) The sinus probably runs anterior to the external carotid artery

10. After elective right carotid endarterectomy (CEA), a patient is noted to have difficulty speaking and is unable to move her left leg while in the recovery room. Which of the following is the most appropriate management of this perioperative neurologic deficit?

(A) Cerebral angiography and admission to the neurology unit
(B) Computed tomography (CT) scan of the head and then intravenous (IV) heparin therapy
(C) Emergent return to the operating room for neck exploration
(D) Admission to the intensive care unit for IV heparin therapy
(E) IV administration of thrombolytic agents (e.g., urokinase)

11. A 25-year-old man was involved in a high-speed motor vehicle accident in which he sustained a right-sided pneumothorax, multiple rib fractures, and a closed, mid-shaft, comminuted tibia fracture. The patient was hemodynamically stable with a Glasgow Coma Scale score of 15 through his trauma evaluation. A chest tube was placed to treat the pneumothorax. Lateral C-spines were negative for fracture, and neurovascular examination was intact preoperatively. The patient was taken to the operating room for intramedullary fixation of the tibia fracture. Postoperatively, during serial neurologic examinations, it was noted that he had some paresthesias and increased pain to his right foot. His toes were cold, with delayed capillary refill. Passive flexion causes significant pain. Which of the following is the most appropriate next step in the management of this patient?

(A) Elevation of the right lower extremity
(B) Compression wrap right lower extremity to reduce swelling
(C) Emergent removal of the intramedullary nail
(D) Measurement of compartment pressures
(E) Increased pain control

12. Three days after an elective esophagectomy for severe esophageal dysplasia a patient is noted to have a worsening left pleural effusion. Which of the following findings in the pleural fluid would most likely suggest injury to the thoracic duct?

(A) Neutrophil count higher than 1000/mL
(B) Glucose = 90 mg/dL
(C) Triglycerides = 200 mg/dL
(D) Red blood cells = 30,000/mL
(E) Specific gravity = 1.010

13. A 56-year-old, white man presents to the emergency department for evaluation of priapism. He admits to taking sildenafil (Viagra) and using a penile injection of prostaglandin at the same time in hopes of improved performance. He takes no other medications. His erection has lasted 4 hours. After aspirating old blood and irrigating with saline he has only a slight detumescence. Which of the following is the most appropriate next step in the management of this patient?

(A) Intracorporal β-adrenergic blockade
(B) Intracorporal α-adrenergic blockade
(C) Angiographic embolization
(D) Intracorporal α-adrenergic agonist
(E) Surgical shunt procedure

14. A 58-year-old man presents to the clinic with a 5-month history of a swelling behind the angle of the mandible on the left side. He has a 100-pack year history of tobacco abuse and drinks a 12-pack of beer a day. He also complains of left ear pain and a sore throat. He is breathing comfortably. Examination of his head and neck reveals a 3-cm firm, slightly tender, fixed mass anterior to his sternocleidomastoid muscle inferior to his mandible and not associated with the parotid gland. His oral cavity shows poor dentition. His nasopharynx and oropharynx are erythematous, but no lesions or masses are found. He has a very strong gag reflex so examination of his larynx is difficult, but no obvious lesions or masses are found. His neck is negative for other masses. Which of the following would be the most appropriate next step in the management of this patient?

(A) Excisional biopsy of the mass in the operating room
(B) Magnetic resonance imaging (MRI) scan of head and neck
(C) Fine needle aspiration (FNA) of the mass
(D) Antibiotic administration and outpatient follow-up
(E) Observation and repeat examination in 6 months

15. A 3-day-old newborn girl is noted to have worsening tachypnea, tachycardia, and failure to thrive. Physical examination demonstrates a harsh, machinery-like, systolic murmur over the precordium. Subsequent echocardiogram reveals a widely patent ductus arteriosus (PDA). Which of the following is the most appropriate management strategy in this infant?

(A) Administration of prostaglandin E_1 (PGE_1)
(B) Emergent ligation of the PDA
(C) Administration of indomethacin
(D) Administration of diuretics
(E) Fluid resuscitation and elective PDA ligation

16. A 70-year-old woman states she "suddenly began to see two of everything next to each other." Examination shows normal vision and pupils of both eyes, however her left eye is turned inward and she is unable to *ab*duct that eye. Which of the following factors associated with this patient's history is most likely unrelated to her current condition?

(A) Hypertension
(B) Diabetes
(C) Strabismus as a child
(D) Recent decrease in hearing
(E) Recent fall

17. A 12-year-old child who complains of a 2-month history of headaches presents with marked diastolic hypertension of 115 mm Hg and a soft bruit heard at the right costovertebral angle. Which of the following is the most likely diagnosis?

(A) Arterial fibrodysplasia
(B) Coarctation of the aorta
(C) Diffuse atherosclerosis
(D) Segmental renal infarction
(E) Chronic ureteral obstruction

18. A 50-year-old woman with a 2-month history of lower back pain that radiates down her right leg comes to your clinic for evaluation. You order a computed tomography (CT) myelogram, which confirms the presence of a herniated disc at the L4–L5 level. The patient wishes to avoid surgery and you initially prescribe conservative treatment with physical therapy. One week later, the patient comes to you with rapidly progressing weakness in her right leg and problems with urinary retention. Which of the following is the next step in this patient's management?

(A) Reassure her that the physical therapy will help and to return to the clinic in 2 weeks if she has not improved
(B) Schedule her for a magnetic resonance imaging (MRI) scan later in the week
(C) Obtain the CT myelogram from 1 week earlier, and take her to the operating room immediately
(D) Tell the patient to stay off her feet for a few days and resume physical therapy when she feels a little better
(E) Admit her to the hospital for observation and inpatient physical therapy

19. A 13-year-old boy presents to the clinic with anterior knee pain on the right. The pain has been present for approximately 2 months. He is an active boy, playing on the basketball and football teams. He has fallen multiple times on his knees, with no serious trauma. He has recently grown in height by 6 inches over the last 4 months. On physical examination, he has pain with resisted extension and direct pressure over the tibial tubercle. Radiographs of the knee show an irregular prominence over the tibia tubercle. Which of the following is most appropriate in the treatment of this patient?

(A) Restriction from serious activity for 4–6 months
(B) Long leg cast application for 8 months
(C) Operative débridement of tibial prominence
(D) Ultrasound therapy to knee
(E) Therapeutic joint aspiration

20. A 3-year-old girl presents to the office with a 3-day history of low-grade fevers, irritability, and left ear pain. She has not had these symptoms before, but has recently recovered from an upper respiratory tract infection. On physical examination she has clear rhinorrhea, the left auricle is normal, and the left external canal is erythematous but not swollen. Her left tympanic membrane is bulging and erythematous, and a middle ear purulent exudate is noted. Her neck has small anterior cervical adenopathy. If a myringotomy is performed and the purulence cultured, which of the following would be the most likely organism cultured?

(A) *Pseudomonas aeruginosa*
(B) *Staphylococcus aureus*
(C) *Streptococcus pneumoniae*
(D) *Bacteroides fragilis*
(E) Herpes simplex virus

21. A 48-year-old woman is postoperative day 12 from an uneventful three-vessel coronary artery bypass surgery for unstable angina. The patient did well postoperatively and was discharged to home on postoperative day 5. The patient states that she began to develop increasing pain around the inferior portion of her incision on postoperative day 9, which became progressively worse and is now associated with yellow, foul-smelling drainage. The patient also notes a 24-hour history of fever, chills, nausea, and vomiting. In the emergency room her temperature is 39° C and her blood pressure is 90/50 mm Hg. Chest computed tomography (CT) reveals significant air and fluid just posterior to the sternal incision. Which of the following is the most appropriate management strategy in this patient?

(A) Administration of oral antibiotics and close outpatient follow-up
(B) Administration of intravenous (IV) antibiotics and percutaneous drainage of the fluid
(C) Opening a small portion of the incision to pack the wound and IV antibiotics
(D) Administration of IV antibiotics and intraoperative sternal débridement
(E) Administration of IV antibiotics and continued inpatient observation

22. A 2-year-old child presents to the office following referral by the pediatrician who has noticed an abdominal mass on routine physical examination. The child has had no symptoms related to the mass. Which of the following characteristics would most likely suggest the diagnosis of a neuroblastoma?

(A) The child also has Beckwith-Wiedemann syndrome
(B) On computed tomography (CT) scan, the tumor has speckled calcifications
(C) On CT scan, the tumor extends into the vena cava
(D) On biopsy, the tumor has blastemal elements, epithelium, and stroma
(E) The patient gives a recent history of hematuria

23. An 18-year-old man is involved in a motor vehicle accident and sustains a T8-level spinal cord injury, resulting in paraplegia. Six months after his accident you are consulted because he has had several febrile urinary tract infections (UTIs). He normally wears a condom catheter. As part of your evaluation, you perform urodynamic testing on the patient. Which type of bladder are you most likely to find?

(A) Spastic bladder
(B) "Mixed-type" bladder
(C) Flaccid bladder
(D) Normal bladder with abnormal external sphincter
(E) Normal bladder with abnormal internal (smooth) sphincter

24. A 42-year-old woman who takes birth control pills presents to the clinic with a recent onset of galactorrhea. A thorough work-up reveals a pituitary adenoma. Which portion of the eye examination may be most revealing?

(A) Extraocular muscle function
(B) Intraocular pressure
(C) Slit-lamp examination
(D) Confrontational visual fields
(E) Retinal examination

25. A 32-year-old beekeeper presents to your office with a 1-month history of seizures and progressive motor weakness. Evaluation reveals a mass on magnetic resonance imaging (MRI), suggestive of astrocytoma. Which of the following is an appropriate statement regarding astrocytomas?

(A) Astrocytomas often cross the corpus callosum, giving a butterfly appearance
(B) Diffuse astrocytomas carry a better prognosis than circumscribed astrocytomas
(C) Diffuse type astrocytomas account for 25% of astrocytomas
(D) Glioblastoma multiforme is associated with a better prognosis than most other astrocytomas
(E) Histologic features include "chicken wire" vasculature and "fried egg" appearance of individual cells

26. A 12-year-old girl presents to the orthopedic clinic because during a routine school screening she was noted to have a possible scoliosis. The patient's mother reports she has not started menstruating. The girl has a normal neurological examination. On forward bending a right thoracic bump was noted. Radiographs reveal a 30° right thoracic curve. Which of the following is the most appropriate next step in the management of this patient?

(A) Observation
(B) Magnetic resonance imaging (MRI)
(C) Physical therapy and exercise regimen
(D) Surgical fusion
(E) Bracing with routine follow-up

27. A 10-year-old boy is playing with a friend, who accidentally hits him in the head with a baseball bat. The boy momentarily loses consciousness, but seems awake and unharmed when his mother finds him. Upon returning home he begins to vomit and mumble incoherently. This clinical picture is most consistent with which of the following?

(A) Acute subdural hematoma
(B) Epidural hematoma
(C) Chronic subdural hematoma
(D) Acute intraventricular hemorrhage
(E) Subarachnoid hemorrhage

28. A 66-year-old woman comes to the clinic with a history of her right eyelid being "droopy." She has a history of hypertension and a 60 pack-year smoking habit. On examination, her right eyelid is 2–3 mm lower than the left. Other findings include normal vision, normal ocular motility, and asymmetric pupils without an afferent pupillary defect. Fundoscopy is normal and she has no other neurologic findings. Which of the following can be most likely ruled out as a cause for this patient's findings?

(A) History of carotid endarterectomy
(B) Lung tumor
(C) Vestibular lesion
(D) Carotid aneurysm
(E) Metastasis to cervical lymph nodes

29. A 35-year-old man is brought to the emergency room after falling 20 feet from the roof of a house. He is noticeably drunk. On examination, his blood pressure is 110/60 mm Hg and his heart rate is 110 beats/min. His abdomen is slightly distended but he denies abdominal tenderness. He has no movement of his lower extremities, no sensation to touch below his umbilicus, but does have voluntary contraction of his anal sphincter and intact proprioception of his lower extremities. Which of the following statements regarding the patient's condition is true?

(A) There is only a 3% chance that this patient will regain any function in the first 24 hours after his injury
(B) A computed tomography (CT) scan of the abdomen and pelvis should be delayed until the cause of the spinal injury is adequately identified
(C) Methylprednisolone should be given within 8 hours and continuously infused over the next 24–48 hours
(D) Radiographs of the thoracic and lumbar spine should be delayed to avoid excessive movement with a suspected C-spine injury
(E) If there is no neck pain on initial examination, the cervical collar may be removed in the emergency room

30. A 35-year-old man sustained a cervical spinal injury in a motor vehicle accident 3 months ago. He has been recovering in a rehabilitation center for several weeks but requires ventilatory support via a tracheostomy tube. During routine suctioning, the patient develops massive bright red bleeding via the tracheostomy tube. Which of the following is the most likely source of this bleeding?

(A) Ruptured arteriovenous malformation with bleeding
(B) Large pulmonary embolus with massive hemoptysis
(C) Pulmonary venous bleeding from pulmonary hypertension
(D) Bleeding from a tracheoinnominate fistula
(E) Bleeding from a tracheoesophageal fistula

31. A 28-year-old man presents to his local primary care physician with a complaint of sudden ringing in his left ear. He awoke 2 days ago and noticed the ringing. He describes it as a high-pitched, continuous ringing that is much worse at night but is always present. He denies otalgia, trauma, headache, dizziness, or recent upper respiratory tract infection. His ear examination is normal. His Weber test lateralizes to the right. Which of the following is the most appropriate next step in the management of this patient with suspected sudden sensorineural hearing loss?

(A) Perform a computed tomography (CT) scan of the head
(B) Administer an antibiotic
(C) Perform an audiogram
(D) Follow-up in 2 weeks for reevaluation
(E) Perform a stapedectomy

32. A 50-year-old man has a 1-year history of documented intermittent claudication but has never developed rest pain or ischemic ulcers. His symptoms have not improved with an exercise program and an attempt at risk-factor management. Arteriography shows a distinct stenosis of the right common iliac artery and normal leg vessels. The patient does not have significant coronary artery disease, and the symptoms are affecting his work performance. Which of the following is the therapy of choice for this patient's claudication?

(A) A weekly aspirin
(B) An aortobifemoral bypass
(C) A right femoropopliteal bypass using saphenous vein
(D) A percutaneous right iliac angioplasty
(E) A right femoral-anterior tibial bypass

33. A 30-year-old woman with headaches, amenorrhea, and galactorrhea is diagnosed with prolactinoma in her pituitary gland. Which of the following statements regarding prolactinomas is true?

(A) These tumors occur only in women
(B) Treatment with bromocriptine can shrink some prolactinomas
(C) Bromocriptine should only be used when surgical removal is not possible
(D) These tumors carry a poor overall prognosis
(E) Prolactinomas are not associated with multiple endocrine neoplasia (MEN) I syndrome

34. A 25-year-old man sustains a severe head injury after a fall from a building. Upon initial evaluation, the patient is noted to have a significant decrease in the level of consciousness and is difficult to arouse. The patient's best response to stimuli includes opening his eyes and drawing up both legs upon sternal rubbing. The patient is also grunting and moaning intermittently. Which of the following best characterizes this patient's Glasgow Coma Scale score?

(A) 5
(B) 6
(C) 7
(D) 8
(E) 9

35. A 39-year-old man gives a 2–3 day history of worsening sensation of "something is in my left eye" accompanied by increasing redness, mild blurring of vision, and mild but worsening pain. Acuity is 20/20 right and 20/40 left. Examination with fluorescein and cobalt blue light reveals a corneal epithelial defect with dendritic extensions. Which of the following is the next most appropriate step in the management of this patient?

(A) Patch the eye with an antibiotic or steroid ointment with follow-up in the eye clinic
(B) Tell the patient he has a sexually transmitted disease and he should inform his partner(s)
(C) Refer the patient to an ophthalmologist for further evaluation
(D) Apply frequent topical antibiotics and follow closely for resolution
(E) Inform the patient he has a herpes zoster virus infection, or "shingles" of the eye

36. A 48-year-old woman presents to the emergency room with seizures. She is noted to have proptosis on physical examination. During her evaluation, a computed tomography (CT) scan is obtained that shows a very large parasagittal mass. Which of the following statements best describes the most likely type of tumor in this patient?

(A) Histology shows psammoma bodies and whorl formation
(B) Five-year survival is less than 20%
(C) These tumors rarely recur after treatment
(D) The tumor cells arise from the dura mater
(E) Chemotherapy is the primary treatment for symptomatic tumors

37. A 30-year-old man involved in a high-speed motor vehicle accident presents to the emergency room awake, but confused. He is hypertensive, tachycardic, and has an obvious left femur fracture and swollen thigh. Chest, pelvis, and lateral C-spine films are negative, as is a head computed tomography (CT) scan. His hematocrit is 21%. Two large-bore intravenous (IV) tubes are placed and lactated Ringer's solution and blood are administered to stabilize the patient. Which of the following is the most appropriate next step in the management of this patient?

(A) Emergent operation for intramedullary nailing of the femur fracture
(B) Skeletal traction to reduce the femur fracture and to tamponade the bone ends
(C) Abdominal computed tomography (CT) or diagnostic peritoneal lavage to rule out intra-abdominal injury
(D) Angiography to the left lower extremity to stop bleeding into the thigh
(E) Continued administration of fluid and observation

Directions: The group of items in this section consists of lettered options followed by a set of numbered items. For each item, select the lettered option(s) that is (are) most closely associated with it. Each lettered option may be selected once, more than once, or not at all.

Questions 38–42

(A) Calcium oxalate
(B) Uric acid
(C) Magnesium ammonium phosphate
(D) Calcium phosphate
(E) Cystine
(F) Calcium carbonate
(G) Xanthine

Match the stone type listed with the most appropriate clinical scenario described below.

38. A 57-year-old man with inflammatory bowel disease who has passed multiple kidney stones over the past 10 years. (SELECT 1 STONE TYPE)

39. A 36-year-old woman has flank pain, microscopic hematuria, and hexagonal crystals in her urine. She has a history of multiple stone-related procedures. (SELECT 1 STONE TYPE)

40. A 29-year-old woman with persistent painless microscopic hematuria and a history of recurrent urinary tract infections (UTIs) that respond to oral therapy, but return after a few weeks to months. (SELECT 1 STONE TYPE)

41. A 44-year-old man with flank pain, hematuria, and a urine pH of 5.0, who says "My kidney stones don't show up on x-rays." (SELECT 1 STONE TYPE)

42. A 22-year-old woman with renal colic and multiple small stones in her kidney on plain radiograph (kidney, ureters, bladder) and a slightly elevated serum calcium. (SELECT 1 STONE TYPE)

Questions 43–47

(A) Esophageal atresia
(B) Congenital cystic adenomatoid malformation (CCAM)
(C) Choanal atresia
(D) Congenital lobar emphysema
(E) Bronchogenic cyst
(F) Foregut duplication
(G) Diaphragmatic hernia
(H) Pulmonary sequestration
(I) Thyroglossal duct cyst

Match each of the following diagnoses with the most appropriate clinical description.

43. A 12-month-old boy presents for evaluation of recurrent "upper respiratory infection." The child has had progressively increasing work of breathing. Chest radiograph shows overexpansion of the left upper lobe. (SELECT 1 DIAGNOSIS)

44. A 2-year-old girl is referred for evaluation of a left lower lobe density noted on a chest radiograph taken for a recent cough. A computed tomography (CT) scan shows a nonaerated segment outside a normal-appearing left lower lobe. A large vessel appears to be feeding the lesion, and arises from below the diaphragm. (SELECT 1 DIAGNOSIS)

45. A 5-year-old girl is referred for evaluation of an abnormal chest radiograph. She has been complaining of nonproductive cough and was found to have a posterior mediastinal cystic mass by computed tomography (CT) scan. Upon resection, the cyst is noted to contain a milky, mucoid fluid, and is lined by columnar epithelium. (SELECT 1 DIAGNOSIS)

46. A newborn boy is admitted to the neonatal intensive care unit for respiratory distress. The chest radiograph shows a cystic lesion in the right middle lobe. A computed tomography (CT) scan shows a microcystic mass limited to the affected lobe, with normal-appearing lung parenchyma surrounding the lesion; vascular anatomy is normal. (SELECT 1 DIAGNOSIS)

47. An 8-year-old boy is referred for evaluation of burning chest pain with developing dysphagia. The child is otherwise healthy. A chest film shows a posterior mediastinal cystic mass. At resection, the cyst is lined by gastric mucosa. (SELECT 1 DIAGNOSIS)

Questions 48–50

(A) Hypoglossal nerve
(B) Ansa hypoglossi
(C) Superior laryngeal nerve
(D) Recurrent laryngeal nerve
(E) Facial vein
(F) Glossopharyngeal nerve
(G) Spinal accessory nerve
(H) Mandibular nerve

Select the appropriate anatomical structure that may account for the patient's signs or symptoms if injured.

48. A 65-year-old man undergoes elective carotid endarterectomy. One week postoperatively, the patient complains that he is having "difficulty speaking." (SELECT 2 STRUCTURES)

49. In the recovery room, the wife of a patient who just underwent carotid endarterectomy notices that her husband's tongue moves toward his neck incision. (SELECT 1 STRUCTURE)

50. In follow-up clinic, a patient who underwent carotid endarterectomy complains of difficulty swallowing. An otorhinolaryngologist performs direct laryngoscopy and notices unilateral vocal cord paralysis. (SELECT 1 STRUCTURE)

Answers and Explanations

1-B. Many patients with coronary artery disease can be treated nonsurgically even in the setting of an acute myocardial infarction (MI). However, there are some settings where surgery is frequently required, such as acute mitral regurgitation caused by ischemic injury to the papillary muscles. At the time of papillary muscle repair the left anterior descending artery (LAD) can also be bypassed surgically, which will decrease the delay in repair of the valve. Angioplasty or administration of tissue plasminogen activator would only delay surgical repair. Mitral valve replacement is generally not required in this setting.

2-D. Meckel diverticulum is a true diverticulum arising in the distal ileum. It commonly presents with painless gastrointestinal bleeding caused by ectopic gastric mucosa. Diagnosis is made by technetium scan for gastric mucosa. Treatment is by excision of the diverticulum. Intussusception may be associated with guaiac-positive stools but typically presents with intermittent abdominal pain, signs and symptoms of small bowel obstruction, and currant jelly stools. Meconium ileus is also associated with signs of obstruction and is primarily seen in neonates. Anal fissure typically presents with severe perianal pain rather than guaiac-positive stools and anemia. Appendicitis does not typically present with melena and anemia.

3-C. This patient's history and physical examination are a typical presentation of idiopathic facial nerve (Bell's) palsy. She is demonstrating a paresis with only weakness and not complete paralysis. This denotes a better prognosis for complete recovery. Electroneurography is reserved for patients with complete paralysis and no evidence of recovery. It is used by some physicians as an indication for surgical decompression. In the setting of suspected malignancy, a computed tomography (CT) scan would be indicated. However, an acute onset of symptoms is more suggestive of an idiopathic process, as opposed to a more progressive weakness, which would indicate a possible malignant-related etiology. Oral steroid therapy may improve recovery from this process and thus is indicated in this setting. Antiviral agents but not antibacterial agents may play a role in the treatment of this process. Heparin may play a role in the treatment of some forms of cerebrovascular disease, but not in the treatment of Bell's palsy.

4-B. A common serious complication associated with supracondylar humeral fractures is development of Volkmann's contracture secondary to compartment syndrome of the forearm. This fracture should be reduced as quickly as possible and immobilized with neurovascular examinations monitored before and after treatment. If compartment syndrome develops, a compartment release may be necessary. Acute respiratory distress syndrome (ARDS) is more frequently associated with large bone fractures and consists of respiratory decompensation and petechiae formation. Growth arrest rarely occurs, but angular deformity may develop in inadequately reduced fractures. Skin breakdown is rare and occurs only if the swelling is not controlled with elevation and prompt reduction of the fracture. The olecranon is part of the ulna and is not at risk for avascular necrosis with this fracture.

5-C. Compartment syndromes are encountered when increased tissue pressure within a limited anatomic space compromises circulation. The most common and most important compartment syndromes occur in relation to interruption and subsequent restoration of blood flow to an extremity made ischemic by an embolism, thrombus, or trauma. The clinical manifestations of compartment syndromes include throbbing and unrelenting pain and the loss of neuromuscular function. Inability to dorsiflex the toes is a grave sign of advanced anterior compartment compression. Treatment for a compartment syndrome is prompt fasciotomy. Electromyographic studies and compartment pressure measurements would probably be abnormal, but are unnecessary in view of the known findings and would delay treatment. Elevation of the leg should accompany fasciotomy but would be ineffective alone. Splinting has no role in the acute management of compression syndromes.

6-B. This patient is suffering from degenerative joint disease of the right hip. She is still quite active. Early management is conservative with nonsteroidal anti-inflammatory drugs (NSAIDs), physical therapy, a cane, and restriction of some activities. If symptoms do not respond to conservative management and activities of daily living are compromised, then elective total hip replacement is an option. Steroid injections may be used as a temporary measure in someone who has severe disease, but this is not considered a first line of treatment. A proximal femoral osteotomy would not be an option because of the patient's age. Radiographs show no lesion, so magnetic resonance imaging (MRI) would not be useful.

7-A. The child most likely has laryngotracheomalacia, which is a syndrome of an immature epiglottic cartilage framework with prolapse of the epiglottis over the airway, causing the symptoms described. In the vast majority of cases the children will do well and grow out of this by 12 months of age. Direct laryngoscopy is often used to make the diagnosis. Infection is unlikely in an afebrile patient in this setting. Tracheostomy is rarely required and is only performed for extremely symptomatic patients in severe respiratory distress. The presenting signs and symptoms and the age of the patient are inconsistent with the diagnosis of a tracheoesophageal fistula, thus an upper gastrointestinal series is not indicated.

8-C. Pericardial cysts most commonly occur at the cardiophrenic angle on the right side. Esophageal duplication cyst is more likely to be found in the posterior mediastinum. Bronchogenic cysts are most likely to be associated with the trachea or right or left bronchi and also would generally not be located in this area. Pulmonary sequestration and cystic bronchogenic carcinoma would more likely be located within the lung parenchyma rather than the central location described.

9-B. The symptoms of a recurrent localized infection with a draining sinus occurring just anterior to the sternocleidomastoid muscle in an infant of this age is consistent with the diagnosis of a persistent second branchial cleft cyst or sinus tract. Sinus tracts of the second branchial cleft typically extend into the tonsillar fossa, passing between the internal and external carotid arteries. Although rare, first branchial cleft cysts may drain into the external auditory canal. Thyroglossal duct cysts are typically midline and may contain thyroid tissue. Persistent branchial cleft cysts are not typically associated with malignancy.

10-C. The primary goal in this situation is to make certain that no technical error has been made during the original operation. The most common technical error is creation of an intimal flap. This can be determined most effectively by immediate neck exploration. Once the neck is opened, the internal carotid artery should be checked for a pulse, a thrill, or intracarotid thrombosis. If the pulse is diminished or there is evidence of thrombosis, the patient should be heparinized and the artery should be reopened to examine for thrombosis or flap elevation. If there are no signs of a carotid problem when the neck is opened, an intraoperative duplex scan or intraoperative arteriogram should be considered to identify intraluminal debris. This is a desperate situation, and angiography, computed tomography (CT) scan, or intensive care admission would only delay the emergent intervention that is necessary. Thrombolytic therapy would not be indicated in patients in the immediate postoperative period.

11-D. This patient is likely developing a compartment syndrome (an increase in pressures in the fascial compartments of his right lower leg). This decreases the blood supply and causes increased pain. Permanent neurovascular and muscle injury can result if the compartment syndrome is not recognized and treated quickly. The pain with passive stretch is classic for compartment syndrome. The initial step may involve measurement of compartment pressures to confirm the diagnosis. Surgical decompression of all compartments is required to prevent further ischemic injury. Elevation of the extremity, placement of a compression wrap, and increased pain control would not address the primary problem and would delay necessary treatment. There would be no need to remove the intramedullary nail in this setting.

12-C. Examination of pleural fluid is often diagnostic in the setting of a chylothorax from an injured thoracic duct. Findings suggestive of a chylothorax include high triglycerides (over 110 mg/dL), high lymphocyte count (400–6800 lymphocytes/(μL), and the presence of chylomicra. Lymphocytes are generally mononuclear, while an elevated neutrophil count is suggestive of an empyema. Red blood cells are nonspecific and may be found in many pleural fluid collections. Normal specific gravity of a chylothorax is 1.012–1.025. Patients with an exudative pleural effusion frequently have a very low glucose level in their pleural fluid, while patients with a transudative effusion (e.g., congestive heart failure) have a higher glucose level (about two-thirds that of serum) within the pleural fluid.

13-D. In nontraumatic cases of priapism like the one described, the goal is to achieve detumescence in under 6 hours to prevent corporal fibrosis. α-Adrenergic agonists like phenylephrine contract smooth muscle and augment detumescence. The other agents listed are ineffective for this purpose. Shunting or embolization is a last resort if pharmacologic manipulation fails.

14-C. In a middle-aged person with significant risk factors for upper aerodigestive tract squamous cell carcinoma, an excisional biopsy of any neck mass is the wrong diagnostic approach. If the mass turns out to be a metastatic lesion, then excisional biopsy may seed the neck with cancer cells. A complete head and neck examination should be performed, and if a suspicious lesion is identified in the upper aerodigestive tract, a biopsy of the lesion should be performed. In addition, a computed tomography (CT) scan should also be performed. The neck should never be violated until cancer is completely ruled out. A magnetic resonance imaging (MRI) scan is not necessary because a good high-quality CT scan is usually adequate for work-up. In the scenario described, a fine needle aspiration (FNA) of the mass should be performed. Prolonged observation would only delay the diagnosis of a potential neoplastic lesion in a patient at significant risk. In addition, evaluation should be performed for high-risk patients before administering any antibiotics.

15-C. The initial treatment of a patent ductus arteriosus (PDA) is attempted closure of the ductus with administration of the prostaglandin inhibitor, indomethacin. Inhibition of prostaglandins results in constriction and closure of the ductus. Indomethacin is frequently effective in newborns although it is generally less effective in full-term infants and children. If newborns do not respond to indomethacin within a week, surgical ligation of the PDA is indicated. Based upon the patient's volume status, diuretics or fluid administration may be required, but these methods do not specifically treat the PDA.

16-C. The most common etiology of abducens (CN VI) palsy is microvascular injury related to hypertension or diabetes. Other considerations include acoustic neuroma, which causes decreased hearing, and basilar skull fracture or increased intracranial pressure as a result of head trauma. A history of strabismus as a child would not be related to this acute onset of misalignment.

17-A. Most asymptomatic children with mildly elevated blood pressure have essential hypertension. However, children with symptoms and a diastolic blood pressure above 100–110 mm Hg usually have secondary hypertension caused by either a renal parenchymal disorder or a renovascular lesion. A common cause of renovascular hypertension in children is arterial fibrodysplasia (fibromuscular dysplasia). It causes about 5%–10% of all cases of renovascular hypertension, and it is primarily a disease of children and premenopausal women. Diffuse atherosclerosis and renovascular hypertension more typically present during the sixth decade of life. Coarctation is usually associated with brachial-femoral pulse discrepancies, and the blood pressure may be high only in one arm. Such hypertension is rarely caused by infarction of the renal parenchyma. Chronic ureteral obstruction is not associated with a bruit at the costovertebral angle.

18-C. When patients with known or suspected disc herniation have progressive motor deficits or symptoms of cauda equina syndrome, emergent surgery is indicated. Any loss of time could be costly, in terms of permanent neurologic deficits. All the other options presented are unacceptable because they ignore the fact that this is a neurologic emergency.

19-A. This patient suffers from tibial apophysitis, or Osgood-Schlatter disease. This typically occurs during the pubertal growth spurt. Evaluation by plain films reveals an enlarged and irregular tibial tubercle with possibly some fracture. Treatment consists of simple restriction from rigorous activities for less severe symptoms. Casting is reserved for severe or refractory cases. Operative débridement is unnecessary in this setting. An ultrasound would not provide additional useful information, and joint aspiration is not therapeutic for this disease.

20-C. The scenario described is most consistent with the diagnosis of acute suppurative otitis media (OM). The most frequently cultured bacteria are *Streptococcus pneumoniae, Haemophilus influenza,* and *Moraxella catarrhalis. Staphylococcus aureus* and *Pseudomonas aeruginosa* are more common in chronic serous OM. Anaerobic bacteria (such as *Bacteroides fragilis*) are rare. The symptoms described are not consistent with herpes zoster oticus.

21-D. Mediastinitis is a rare but serious complication of patients undergoing surgery via a median sternotomy. Patients at particular risk are those undergoing coronary artery bypass grafting (CABG) with utilization of both internal mammary arteries. Appropriate treatment involves administration of intravenous (IV) antibiotics, appropriate fluid resuscitation, and intraoperative surgical débridement of infected tissue including the sternum. Percutaneous fluid drainage or simple packing of the skin wound would not provide adequate débridement of tissue. Observation or outpatient follow-up would be inappropriate.

22-B. Neuroblastoma is the most common tumor in newborns and arises from neural crest cells anywhere from the neck to the pelvis. A characteristic finding on radiographs of neuroblastoma is speckled calcifications mixed in the parenchyma of the tumor. In addition, neuroblastomas may be associated with increased urinary levels of homovanillic acid (HVA) and vanillylmandelic acid (VMA). Wilms tumor, not neuroblastoma, is associated with Beckwith-Wiedemann syndrome, hemihypertrophy, and Drash syndrome; may extend into the inferior vena cava; and is generally composed of blastemal elements, epithelium, and stroma. In addition, Wilms tumor may be associated with hematuria, unlike neuroblastoma.

23-A. Lesions of the spinal cord above the sacral micturition center (T12) cause bladder spasticity. Lesions below and damage to nerves cause bladder flaccidity. This patient is most likely having infections because of inadequate urine drainage and possibly elevated intravesical pressures, which might be treated with clean catheterization and anticholinergic medications to reduce intravesical pressures.

24-D. Pituitary tumors can compress the optic chiasm, resulting in bitemporal visual field defects. This can be tested by confrontational visual fields testing. One would not expect the other aspects of the eye examination to be affected.

25-A. Diffuse astrocytomas are the most common type, accounting for 75% of all astrocytomas. They carry a much poorer prognosis than the circumscribed type. On computed tomography (CT) scan these tumors cross the corpus callosum, giving a characteristic butterfly appearance. Glioblastoma multiforme is the most common diffuse astrocytoma and carries a dismal prognosis. "Chicken wire" vasculature and "fried egg" appearance of cells is characteristic of oligodendrogliomas, not astrocytomas.

26-E. The patient has idiopathic adolescent scoliosis. The greatest chance of progression of a scoliotic curve is during the pubertal growth spurt. It appears that this patient has a correctable growth as she has not started menses. Bracing and follow-up every 4–6 months is necessary to monitor for curve progression. If the curve progresses to greater than 45° despite bracing, surgical fusion may be necessary. Magnetic resonance imaging (MRI) is not necessary in idiopathic adolescent scoliosis if the patient has a normal neurologic examination. Observation alone would not be adequate, and physical therapy without bracing would also not adequately treat the abnormal curvature.

27-B. The child has a history that is classic for epidural hematoma. He sustained a hard blow in the region of the middle meningeal artery, which is the source of bleeding in 85% of epidural hematomas. He also had the classic clinical course of loss of consciousness, followed by a "lucid interval," followed by neurologic deterioration and nausea or vomiting. Both acute and chronic subdural hematomas are more common in the elderly and usually result from tearing of a bridging vessel after acceleration/deceleration of the brain. Both traumatic intraventricular hemorrhage and subarachnoid hemorrhage are possible, but the history is much more suggestive of epidural bleeding. In addition, epidural hematomas require urgent surgical intervention and therefore must be ruled out. A computed tomography (CT) scan of the head should confirm the diagnosis.

28-C. Horner syndrome results from injury to the sympathetic fibers leading to the pupil, causing a parasympathetic miosis (small pupil). The pathway begins in the hypothalamus and synapses in the ciliospinal center of Budge between C8 and T2, then to synapse in the superior cervical ganglion after passing the lung apex, and tracks with the internal carotid artery into the skull. Potential causes of injury to this tract include apical lung tumors, iatrogenic injuries (i.e., with carotid endarterectomy), carotid aneurysms, and cervical lymph node disease. Vestibular lesions would not be associated with such findings.

29-C. Only 3% of patients with a complete spinal cord injury (SCI) will regain any function in the first 24 hours. The patient described has an incomplete injury, as evidenced by sacral sparing and intact proprioception. Management of SCIs should include methylprednisolone within the first 8 hours and continued for 24–48 hours. Radiographs of the entire spine should be taken to elucidate sites of injury, and the systolic blood pressure should be maintained at higher than 90 mm Hg, with adequate oxygenation. Furthermore, despite the obvious neurologic deficit, this patient should undergo a thorough evaluation for other potential life-threatening injuries without delay. In this case, a computed tomography (CT) scan of the abdomen would be appropriate to rule out potential intra-abdominal or pelvic injuries. A thorough evaluation of the cervical spine is warranted in every SCI. Stabilization of the C-spine is very important in the prevention of further neurologic damage. In patients with an impaired sensorium (i.e., excessive alcohol use), the lack of neck pain on physical examination may be unreliable in the assessment of patients with potential C-spine injuries, and should not be relied upon for criteria for removal of the cervical collar.

30-D. A tracheoinnominate fistula is rare but may present in patients with a chronically indwelling endotracheal tube or tracheostomy tube with a high-pressure balloon cuff. Most cuffs today are high volume and low pressure to avoid exceeding tracheal capillary pressure with resulting ischemia. Sudden massive onset of bright red bleeding from the tracheostomy tube is a characteristic presentation. Pulmonary emboli do not present with hemoptysis but rather respiratory distress and cardiovascular collapse. The patient's history is not consistent with arteriovenous malformation or the development of pulmonary hypertension.

31-C. Tinnitus is a common symptom of sudden sensorineural hearing loss. The Weber test lateralizes to the better hearing ear with a sensorineural hearing loss and to the worse hearing ear with a conductive hearing loss. In this setting, an immediate audiogram is indicated to diagnose hearing loss. If hearing loss is present, then immediate treatment with oral steroids is indicated to improve the chance for recovery. Antiviral medications, but not antibacterial agents, are often given along with the steroids because of the theory of a possible viral etiology. For steroids to have maximal benefit, immediate treatment is indicated and a 2-week waiting period is too long. A head computed tomography (CT) scan is not indicated. A head magnetic resonance imaging (MRI) scan may be indicated in patients with a suspected acoustic neuroma, although dizziness is generally a common symptom in patients with such a lesion. There is no indication for a stapedectomy in this setting.

32-D. Balloon angioplasty is especially effective for localized, short stenotic lesions or short-length occlusions of the iliac arteries, with about 90% initial recanalization and long-term patency of 60%–70% at 4 years. Femoropopliteal and femoral-anterior tibial bypass are unnecessary because this patient's superficial femoral and popliteal arteries are not diseased. The patient's left iliac system is not stenotic and therefore an aortobifemoral bypass is unnecessary. Daily aspirin reduces overall vascular mortality rate by 15% and apparently benefits the patency of vascular repairs, especially if the drug is begun preoperatively.

33-B. Prolactinomas can occur in both men and women. Bromocriptine, a dopamine agonist, is the first line treatment of symptomatic prolactinomas. Bromocriptine should also be started if prolactin levels are higher than 500. Bromocriptine is often successful at arresting the growth of prolactinomas, and can sometimes shrink the tumors. Surgery is indicated if bromocriptine therapy fails. Prolactinomas may be associated with multiple endocrine neoplasia (MEN) I syndrome. The overall prognosis of these tumors is excellent.

34-D. The Glasgow Coma Scale (GSC) is commonly used to standardize the evaluation of patients with a head injury or a decreased level of consciousness. Sternal rubbing is used to produce a painful stimulus in patients with a decreased level of consciousness. Only opening the eyes to painful stimuli is counted as 2 points, while withdrawing to painful stimuli without localization is 4 points. Incomprehensible sounds represents a verbal response score of 2. Thus this patient has a GCS score of $2 + 4 + 2 = 8$.

35-C. A corneal epithelial defect with dendritic extensions is typical for a herpes simplex type 1 infection on the cornea. It is **not** related to sexual contact. Topical steroids can make the infection worse and result in corneal ulceration. Treatment includes topical antiviral drops and ophthalmologic evaluation.

36-A. This patient's history is suggestive of meningioma. Psammoma bodies and whorl formation are characteristic of the histology of these tumors. Meningiomas arise from the arachnoid cells, not the dura mater. These lesions are followed closely and when symptomatic the treatment of choice is surgical excision. Smaller lesions may be amenable to high-dose, focused beam radiation (gamma knife). Although benign, meningiomas do commonly recur after excision.

37-C. Although a femur fracture can result in significant blood loss, intra-abdominal injury must be ruled out before the femur fracture can be addressed. Trauma evaluation should be completed, and in a patient who is hypertensive, a diagnostic peritoneal lavage or computed tomography (CT) scan of the abdomen should be done as quickly as possible to rule out intra-abdominal injury that may be life-threatening. A femur fracture can be quickly placed in a traction splint to provide comfort while the patient undergoes the trauma evaluation. Emergent intramedullary nailing or performance of angiography should not precede evaluation for potential intra-abdominal injuries. Observation alone with fluid administration would not be appropriate in this situation.

38-A. Gut calcium complexes with fats and leaves oxalate unbound. Excess oxalate is then absorbed and excreted in the urine, causing these stones. Treatment is hydration and avoidance of oxalate-rich foods.

39-E. Hexagonal crystals are pathognomonic for cystine lithiasis. These hard stones often require multiple treatments. Treatment is with increased fluid intake and drugs (e.g., d-penicillamine, mercaptopropionylglycine).

40-C. Struvite (magnesium ammonium phosphate) stones are often seen in this setting of frequent urinary tract infections (UTIs) due to urease-producing bacteria. Treatment is complete stone removal, urinary acidification, and urease inhibitors (e.g., acetohydroxamic acid).

41-B. Uric acid stones tend to form in an acidic (low pH) urine, as the pKa of uric acid is 5.5. Alkalinization is often helpful in prevention and dissolution of existing stones.

42-D. This scenario of multiple stones in a young woman should raise suspicion of hyperparathyroidism and this diagnosis must be ruled out. Calcium phosphate stones are commonly seen in this setting. Serum calcium is the best single test to screen for hyperparathyroidism.

43-D. Congenital lobar emphysema is an overexpansion of a segment of lung parenchyma. It occurs because of abnormal cartilaginous bronchi, which allow airway collapse and air trapping. The overexpansion may be progressive and may lead to mediastinal shift and cardiorespiratory failure. Diagnosis is made by plain chest radiograph, and treatment is by resection of the affected lobe.

44-H. Pulmonary sequestration is a pulmonary anomaly that has no communication with the tracheobronchial tree. The lesion may present with respiratory compromise, but more commonly is diagnosed by abnormal chest radiograph obtained for mild respiratory symptoms. The lesion may be intralobar (wholly contained within a normal pulmonary lobe) or extralobar (completely outside the normal parenchyma). Intralobar lesions are usually isolated lesions, whereas extralobar lesions are frequently associated with other anomalies. The most significant finding is the presence of anomalous vascular supply. Pulmonary sequestration frequently has anomalous feeding vessels that most commonly arise directly from the aorta, often below the diaphragm.

45-E. Bronchogenic cyst is a posterior mediastinal cystic mass that usually does not produce symptoms until it reaches a size large enough to compress surrounding structures. The mass is noticed on plain chest radiograph and is further defined by computed tomography (CT) scan. The cyst is lined by cuboidal or columnar epithelium, and is filled with a milky fluid. Treatment is by excision.

46-B. Congenital cystic adenomatoid malformation (CCAM) is a pulmonary anomaly characterized by the development of bronchial structures at the expense of alveolar development. Cystic parenchyma results, and may be microcystic or macrocystic in nature. Clinical presentation may vary from mild to severe respiratory distress, or may be asymptomatic until recurrent infection develops. Treatment is by resection because of the risk of recurrent infection. Fetal hydrops may be associated with CCAM, and the combination is associated with a high mortality rate (90%).

47-F. Foregut duplication presents as a posterior mediastinal cystic mass and may be difficult to differentiate from bronchogenic cyst. Clues to the diagnosis may be related to the frequent presence of ectopic gastric mucosa, with resultant ulceration and possible bleeding. The cyst may rupture, leading to diagnosis with pleural effusion. The computed tomography (CT) scan findings are similar to bronchogenic cyst. At resection, these cysts are filled with a clear or bloody fluid, and are lined with gastric mucosa.

48-C and D. The rich supply of vessels and nerves in the neck requires a thorough knowledge of the anatomy of this area and precise operative technique if injuries are to be avoided when performing carotid endarterectomy. Superior laryngeal nerve dysfunction can cause easy fatigability of the voice, while unilateral injury to the recurrent laryngeal nerve can cause hoarseness. Obtaining a thorough description of the patient's complaint of "difficulty speaking" is important in directing the evaluation and treatment of this patient.

49-A. The hypoglossal nerve crosses the carotid artery 1–2 cm cephalad to its bifurcation. Injury to it will result in deviation of the tongue to the side of the operation.

50-D. The recurrent laryngeal nerve injury can cause vocal cord paralysis, hoarseness, and minor swallowing difficulty. Injury to both the left and right recurrent laryngeal nerves can cause bilateral vocal cord paralysis and severe respiratory distress secondary to obstruction of the airway at the level of the vocal cords. This is a medical emergency requiring prompt diagnosis and airway control.

Index